HANDBOOK OF GENITOURINARY MEDICINE

NEW RESEARCH

RENAL AND UROLOGIC DISORDERS

Additional books in this series can be found on Nova's website
under the Series tab.

Additional e-books in this series can be found on Nova's website
under the e-book tab.

HANDBOOK OF GENITOURINARY MEDICINE

NEW RESEARCH

RASHMI R. SINGH
EDITOR

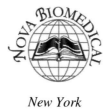

New York

For permission to use material from this book please contact us:
Telephone 631-231-7269; Fax 631-231-8175
Web Site: http://www.novapublishers.com

NOTICE TO THE READER

The Publisher has taken reasonable care in the preparation of this book, but makes no expressed or implied warranty of any kind and assumes no responsibility for any errors or omissions. No liability is assumed for incidental or consequential damages in connection with or arising out of information contained in this book. The Publisher shall not be liable for any special, consequential, or exemplary damages resulting, in whole or in part, from the readers' use of, or reliance upon, this material. Any parts of this book based on government reports are so indicated and copyright is claimed for those parts to the extent applicable to compilations of such works.

Independent verification should be sought for any data, advice or recommendations contained in this book. In addition, no responsibility is assumed by the publisher for any injury and/or damage to persons or property arising from any methods, products, instructions, ideas or otherwise contained in this publication.

This publication is designed to provide accurate and authoritative information with regard to the subject matter covered herein. It is sold with the clear understanding that the Publisher is not engaged in rendering legal or any other professional services. If legal or any other expert assistance is required, the services of a competent person should be sought. FROM A DECLARATION OF PARTICIPANTS JOINTLY ADOPTED BY A COMMITTEE OF THE AMERICAN BAR ASSOCIATION AND A COMMITTEE OF PUBLISHERS.

Additional color graphics may be available in the e-book version of this book.

Library of Congress Cataloging-in-Publication Data

ISBN: 978-1-62618-226-4

Library of Congress Control Number: 2013933188

Published by Nova Science Publishers, Inc. † New York

Contents

Preface

Genitourinary tract consists of organs of the urinary tract as well as the reproductive tract. Disorders of the genitourinary system include a range of disorders from those that are asymptomatic to those that manifest an array of signs and symptoms. Causes for these disorders include congenital anomalies, infectious diseases, trauma, malignancy or conditions that secondarily involve the urinary structure. Advancement of scientific technologies such as genomic and/ or proteomic arrays, single nucleotide polymorphisms, sequencing, etc have enabled these organs to be studied extensively. A lot of information is now accumulating on the genes, gene mutations and their products to be analyzed and their biological and pathological role in the disease. Prostate, Renal and Bladder cancer incidences are increasing and there is a growing need to identify potential genes and target the disease with novel molecules so as to suppress/shrink the growth of these tumor cells. Tissue engineering is a latest technology whereby, the use of a combination of cells, engineering and materials methods, and suitable biochemical and physio-chemical factors are used to improve or replace biological functions.

Hence, as an Editor, I feel privileged to have been given an opportunity to present a handbook that is a compilation of all recent advances and updates on genitourinary medicine and research. The book comprises of chapters that include research review papers on role of matrix metalloproteinases in urothelial cancers, epigenetic mechanisms in urogenital cancers, role of toll-like receptor genes in prostate cancers, use of model models to understand genitourinary malformations and clinical papers that describe the role of chemotherapy in bladder cancers, emerging novel treatments in renal cell carcinoma, clinical management of patients with Vesicoureteric reflux and tissue engineering to restore tissues of the genitourinary tract. A special chapter is included to understand the role of specific gene/s and their mutations in the development of Pediatric nephritic syndromes.

Each chapter is written by researchers and clinicians with expertise in their field. The authors not only provide extensive literature review, but also summarize personal research findings and clinical experience. The book would be most useful to not only clinicians, surgeons and physicians, but also researchers, research fellows and scientists who are deeply involved in understanding genitourinary diseases. We personally hope that readers will be motivated to reading this book.

I would once again sincerely thank each and every author for providing their valuable time to contribute to this handbook. I would also like to acknowledge the entire staff at Nova Publishers for haven given me this opportunity and for their timely help and support.

Rashmi Singh

Dr Rashmi R Singh, *Ph.D.*
Scientific and Clinical Consultant,
SciReg Pharma,
Vancouver, BC, Canada.

In: Handbook of Genitourinary Medicine: New Research   ISBN: 978-1-62618-226-4
Editor: Rashmi R. Singh   © 2013 Nova Science Publishers, Inc.

Chapter I

Emerging Trends in the Treatment of Kidney Cancers

Rashmi R. Singh and Ravibhushan Singh
SciReg Pharma, Vancouver, BC, Canada

Abstract

Kidney cancers or renal cell carcinomas (RCC's) constitute a heterogeneous group of primary epithelial tumors of the kidney with malignant potential. This disease displays relative resistance to radiation and chemotherapy, although occasional durable responses to interleukin-2-based immunotherapy have been observed. However, radical nephrectomy is still the gold standard for larger and central tumors. The identification, characterization and pathogenetic role of the von-Hippal Lindau (*VHL*) gene in 1993 in conventional RCC (cRCC) led to the discovery of bevacizumab; a humanized monoclonal antibody targeting vascular endothelial growth factor (*VEGF*) that is normally regulated by *VHL*, but is over expressed when *VHL* gene is mutated. On a similar line, some of the recent emerging therapeutic developments in the treatment of RCC include agents that target angiogenesis (sunitinib and pazopanib) and a mammalian target of rapamycin (mTOR) targeted therapy, and temsirolimus have been approved as front-line agents. Sorafenib and sunitinib have shown antitumor activity as first- and second-line therapy in patients with cytokine-refractory metastatic RCC who have conventional/clear-cell histology. These agents have largely replaced cytokines (immunotherapy) in treatment-naive patients. This chapter summarizes some of the recently identified molecules, some of which are currently at the clinical phase of testing the treatment of advanced stage RCC.

Introduction

Urological malignancies include malignancies affecting urinary tract and constitute a large portion of work load of urologists. Genitourinary diseases involve disorders of the genital and urinary organs such as the prostate, bladder, kidney, testis, and penis. Genitourinary diseases can be classified as either benign or malignant. Testicular cancer is most common in young men between 20 and 35 years of age. In contrast, the highest incidence of kidney cancer and bladder cancer is in adults between 60 and 70 years of age. Prostate cancer is the most common genitourinary malignancy in men and the incidence of prostate cancer increases with age. There are many genetic, racial, environmental, and behavioral risk factors that contribute to development of genitourinary malignancies. Cigarette smoking is the most significant risk factor, and smokers have shown to be at a four-fold higher risk. Historical developments in the management of genitourinary malignancies are similar to the developments in other cancers. Surgery was the only treatment possible until the beginning of the 20th century, when radiation therapy became available [1].

With the advent of novel molecular technologies that allow a thorough investigation of genetic and protein changes leading to the initiation, promotion, formation, and progression of tumors, genitourinary malignancies are now being researched at their most fundamental level.

Kidney Carcinomas: Renal Cell Carcinoma (RCC)

Epidemiology and Incidence of RCC

Kidney cancers are also more commonly called as Renal Cell Carcinoma (RCC). They are defined as a heterogeneous group of sporadic or hereditary carcinomas derived from the epithelial cells of the kidneys with malignant potential. These tumors account for around 3% of the total adult malignancies [2, 3]. The incidence continues to grow with incidental discoveries of small renal masses.

Despite improvements in the management of localized RCC, most patients are diagnosed with advanced RCC, which is often refractory and associated with a poor prognosis [4]. 90-95% of the neoplasms that arise from the renal cortex of the kidney are parenchymal in origin [3]. The sporadic form of the disease occurs at a very late age in life around 50-70 yrs with median age of diagnosis of around 65 years. The disease is usually associated with formation of unilateral /solitary renal tumors with rare incidence in children below the age of 3 yrs, while the hereditary forms occur earlier in life and are associated with formation of multifocal, bilateral tumors. The etiology of RCC is still not known although a large number of hormonal, genetic, environmental and cellular factors have shown to be associated with the disease [5].

This disease is characterized by lack of early warning signs, diverse clinical manifestations, relative resistance to radiation and chemotherapy [6]. Surgical resection by radical nephrectomy is considered to be the only effective and gold standard treatment in the localized form of kidney cancer, yet, even in this case, 20–30% of patients will still experience recurrence of the disease [7]. Radiotherapy is generally used when surgery is not a suitable option for many patients.

Metastatic renal cell carcinoma is highly resistant to chemotherapeutic agents and thus multiple agents, including hormone therapy, radiation, and immune therapy, have been tried, and none have produced effective benefits [8].

Immuno-Cytokine Therapy: A Conventional Remedy

Immune therapy with cytokines has been the most conventional treatment options for patients with advanced disease. The cytokines are an important family of BRMs (biologic response modulators) that include Interleukin-2 (IL-2) and Interferons. Used either alone or in combination, they have represented the first line of treatment of kidney cancer.

Recombinant Interleukin-2 (rIL-2) or *Proleukin* is a BRM available for the treatment of advanced kidney cancer [9]. The first indication that IL-2 could induce a response in metastatic RCC patients was first reported in 1985 [10] and was later approved by FDA in 1992. It is known to be a potent immune stimulator with some anti-angiogenic activity. It stimulates the growth of T cells and "natural killer" (NK) white blood cells. T cells are very important in body's fight against cancer because they recognize cancer cells and set off an alarm to the body. The NK cells respond to this alarm and are transformed into lymphokine-activated killer (LAK) cells, which are capable of destroying cancer cells [11]. (Kidney Cancer Association, *www.KidneyCancer.org*).

Interferons are widely used to treat kidney cancer, either alone or in combination with other drugs. Interferon is in very common use for kidney cancer in the US, and in many countries, it is the only standard therapy or close to that. Like Interleukin-2, Interferon is a cytokine and is manufactured as a drug through genetic engineering techniques. There are several different classes of interferons, however, only Interferon-Alpha (IFN-α) is commonly used to treat kidney cancer. There are two slightly different alpha-interferons used to treat kidney cancer, Interferon-Alpha-2a, trade name Roferon, and Interferon-Alpha-2b, trade name Intron-A. There is no major difference between these drugs. Interferon works differently than IL-2. It acts by making the tumor cells more susceptible to immune attack by increasing the degree to which they present antigen on their surface. If the immune system recognizes these antigens as abnormal, then it may be able to attach and destroy the cells. It also has a modest direct effect on growth of the cancer cells themselves. It can apparently also stimulate some immune cells such as Natural Killer (NK) Cells [11].

Immuno therapy with cytokines has always been the first line of treatment for patients with metastatic disease associated with a prolonged survival only in a subset of patients [4]. IL-2 when used alone has shown a response rate of 7-23%, almost similar to IFN-a, with one-third being complete remissions. However, only 10%–20% of patients experienced objective disease response [12, 13, 14, 15]. Escudier et al. [15] in their studies have revealed worst results and poor responses (<5%) when patients were treated with other cytokines (e.g. interferon following high-dose IL-2 failure) as a second- line of treatment. On the contrary, both IL-2 and IFN-α are associated with significant toxicity [16] and thus not well tolerated in patients.

Kidney Cancer Is Heterogeneous

RCC is not a single disease, but it has several morphological subtypes. RCC's are considered to be histologically, clinically and genetically a very heterogeneous group of tumors. This heterogeneity has been a controversy for a long time in the clinical diagnosis of RCC. There have been important advances in the knowledge of the genetic basis of RCC. Genetic abnormalities for each of the pathological types have been identified and are considered to be unique signatures for each subtype [17]. Since the oncogenic mechanisms are unique for each subtype, there exist distinct disease specific approaches to therapy. The malignant renal tumors of conventional or classical clear-cell renal cell carcinoma (cRCC) histology accounts for 85% of total surgical cases. This tumor type was shown to be highly associated with the *VHL* tumor suppressor gene that was first identified and characterized in 1993 [18]. The *VHL* gene was shown to be mutated both in hereditary RCC as well as in most cases of sporadic clear-cell RCC, the former due to a germline mutation of one allele and loss of heterozygosity of the other, and the latter due to acquired mutations in both alleles [19]. *VHL* gene has demonstrated its role in the regulation of gene transcription, the regulation of oxygen-dependent genes and their expression and the control of tumor angiogenesis via the vascular endothelial growth factor (*VEGF*) [20].

Unfortunately, despite substantial knowledge of its genetics and identification of key signaling pathways, both incidence and mortality of RCC have steadily worsened over the last several decades.

von Hippal Lindau (VHL) in cRCC

The functions of the *VHL* gene and pVHL have been extensively elucidated. The biology of the *VHL* gene and its role continues to be unraveled as the molecular mechanisms by which pVHL modulates the expression of target genes in cRCC's are now being investigated. A role has been demonstrated in the regulation of gene transcription, the regulation of oxygen-dependent genes and their expression and the control of tumor angiogenesis via the vascular endothelial growth factor (*VEGF*) [20]. The transcription of *VEGF* and erythropoietin (EPO) genes is a phenomenon characteristic of hypoxic tissues, known as hypoxia-inducible genes, such as hypoxia-inducible factor or *HIF* [21]. It is now known that hypoxia-inducible factors HIF1a and HIF2a are substrates of pVHL and are potent inducers of angiogenic and growth factor peptides. In normal cells, HIF-1a subunits accumulate under hypoxic conditions, combine with HIF-1b subunits and cause accumulation of proteins, which ultimately provide valuable protection from the effects of chronic hypoxia. Activated HIF leads to the transcription of several genes whose corresponding proteins are important for blood vessel growth and oxygen delivery, such as VEGF, erythropoietin, platelet-derived growth factor (PDGF) and transforming growth factor-a (TGF-a). Hence, RCC's are highly angiogenic tumors. Recent studies have also demonstrated the role in regulation of extra cellular pH [22], formation of extra cellular matrix [23] and cell cycle control [24]. Poorer overall survival and progression-free survival have been reported in patients with loss of function mutations [25], although a much larger study found *VHL* mutation or methylation to be strongly associated with better prognosis in Stage I to III patients but not in Stage IV patients [26].

With the *VHL* gene functions studied so extensively and the high angiogenic phenotype of tumors associated with VHL disease, novel therapeutic approaches involving the inhibition of HIF thereby targeting this pathway are being explored as a way to develop specific therapy for a causative mutation [16, 27].

This chapter briefly summarizes and highlights some of the novel interventions and treatment modalities that could provide a more positive outlook for the future management of metastatic RCC and possibly an increase in the overall survival of patients.

Novel Targeted Therapies in RCC

In recent years, clinical trials have established the role of targeted therapy as the first line of therapy in patients with metastatic disease. An increased understanding of the *VHL* gene pathway has led to the development of drugs which have demonstrated the ability to shrink the tumor in patients with advanced cRCC. Some of the current targeted therapies for cRCC include monoclonal antibodies and targeting the genes that are regulated by *VHL* gene and transcriptionally upregulated by HiFs (hypoxia- inducible factors) such as those coding for *VEGF* (vascular endothelial growth factor), *VEGF* receptors, the *PDGF* (platelet derived growth factor) receptor, tyrosine kinase inhibitors and the serine–threonine protein kinase mammalian target of rapamycin (mTOR)–HiF pathway. Of these, *VEGF* is one of the most promising of the anti-angiogenesis targets. Some of the targeted therapies currently under trials for potential RCC treatment are listed in Table 1.

Table 1. Summarizes some of the novel targeted therapies used as treatment modalities in advanced RCC

Target genes	Therapeutic Agents	Mechanism of action
VEGF	Bevacizumab (Avastin)	Humanized antibody to *VEGF*
VEGFR1, VEGFR2	VEGF trap	Receptors fused to IgG1-Fc
Raf, VEGF, PDGF	BAY 43-9006 (Nexavar, Sorafenib tosylate)	Kinase inhibitor
VEGFR2, PDGFR, c-Kit, Fms-like tyrosine kinase 3	SU11248 (Sutent, sunitinib malate)	Tyrosine kinase inhibitor
EGFR	ZD1839 (Iressa)	Tyrosine kinase inhibitor
EGFR	OSI-774 (Tarceva, erlotinib)	Tyrosine kinase inhibitor
EGFR	C-225 (Erbitux, Cetuximab)	Humanized Ab to *EGFR*
VEGFR1,2,3 PDGFR, c-Kit, Fms-like tyrosine kinase 3, (*IYK*), (*Lck*)	Votrient (Pazopanib)	Multi targeted Tyrosine Kinase Inhibitor
VEGFR1,2,3 PDGFR, c-Kit	Inlyta (Axitinib)	Small molecule tyrosine kinase Inhibitor
VEGF Pathway	Tivozanib (Aveo)	Tyrosine Kinase Inhibitor
HIF-1	Topotecan, others	Topoisomerase I poison Small molecule inhibitors
mTOR	Torisel (Temsirolimus) Afinitor (Everolimus)	mTOR pathway
p21	Antisense oligo- RAD001 (everolimus)	Promote apoptosis after DNA damage

EGFR, epidermal growth factor receptor; *VEGF*, vascular endothelial growth factor; *HIF*, hypoxia-inducible factor; *PDGF*, platelet-derived growth, *IYK*, Interleukin-2 receptor inducible T-cell kinase; *Lck*, Leukocyte-specific protein tyrosine kinase; *mTOR*, mammalian target of rapamycin.

Monoclonal Antibodies

Monoclonal antibodies are functionally designed to attach to particular sites on a tumor and to deliver anti-cancer drugs to the tumor with great specificity. Bevacizumab (trade name Avastin) was FDA-approved for kidney cancer in August 2009. It was the first commercially available antibody that was designed to specifically bind to a VEGF protein that plays an important role throughout the lifecycle of the kidney tumor to develop and maintain blood vessels, a process known as angiogenesis. Bevacizumab exerts its action by interfering with the blood supply to the tumor by directly binding to the VEGF protein to prevent interactions with receptors on blood vessel cells [16]. Yang JC et al. [28] in their phase II trial with clear-cell RCC who had metastatic disease revealed progression, prolonged overall survival, but there was no significant improvement in survival. A phase III trial of IFN-α or IFN-α plus bevacizumab in metastatic RCC is underway [7, 29].

Tyrosine Kinase Inhibitors (TKI)

Many growth factor receptors require phosphorylation on tyrosine residues by the so-called 'tyrosine kinases' in order for them to become activated and convey their signals to the cellular replicative machinery. This was the basis for the development of a group of tyrosine kinase inhibitors two of which were approved by the FDA in 2005 and 2006. These were sorafenib tosylate (Nexavar) and sunitinib malate (Sutent). Both of these new drugs disrupt the angiogenesis process. Sorafenib and sunitinib have shown antitumor activity as first- and second-line therapy in patients with cytokine-refractory metastatic RCC who have conventional/ clear-cell histological features. Although complete responses are not common, both drugs promote disease stabilization and increase progression-free survival [30].

Sorafenib (Sorafenib Tosylate)

Also known as Nexavar, Sorafenib was approved by the FDA in December 2005 for the treatment of advanced metastatic RCC. Sorafenib imparts its action by targeting blood supply of a tumor, depriving it of the oxygen and nutrients needed for growth. The molecular targets of sorafenib include the tyrosine kinases VEGFR-2 and-3, PDGFR-b, FLT3, KIT and RET, and the serine/threonine Raf kinases, B-Raf and Raf-1/C-Raf. [11, 16, 30]. By blocking VEGF, platelet-derived growth factor (PDGF) and Raf-kinase pathway, Sorafenib can interfere with the tumor cell's ability to increase its blood supply, tumor cell growth and proliferation. Clinical studies also indicate that it can significantly slow tumor progression [11].

Sutent (Sunitinib Malate)

Sutent was discovered a month after Nexavar and is used as a second- line of treatment of RCC. Sunitinib is shown to exhibit a higher potency against advanced RCC, perhaps because it inhibits more receptors than sorafenib. Sutent is a tyrosine kinase inhibitor that is similar to Gleevec in some ways. Sutent also inhibits the "VEGF" receptors. Sutent deprives tumor cells of the blood and nutrients needed to grow by interfering with VEGF and PDGF signaling pathways. Sutent was approved by the FDA in 2006 for kidney cancer patients because of its ability to reduce the size of tumors [11]. Clinical studies have also showed a favorable response rate in patients with metastatic kidney cancer whose tumors had progressed following immunotherapy. In a Phase III study comparing Sutent with IFN-α, Sutent offered a superior efficacy compared to IFN-α, with a double progression-free survival, a benefit in patients with poor prognosis at baseline studies, tumor shrinkage in around 28% patients and a better quality of life compared to patients treated with IFN-α [31].

Recent clinical studies formed the basis for new guidelines for the treatment of advanced RCC: sorafenib should be used as a second-line treatment, sunitinib as the first-line therapy for good and intermediate-risk patients [32].

Except for side effects such as hand-foot syndrome, rash, fatigue, hypertension, and diarrhea, sorafenib and sutent are potential drugs for treatment of advanced RCC [11, 16, 30, 32].

ZD1839 (Iressa)

Iressa in a Phase II trial did not show anti-tumor activity at the doses and schedules studied [33]. In contrast, *erlotinib* when used in combination with avastin (bevacizumab) shows comparatively a better effect than when used alone [7].

Votrient (Pazopanib)

Votrient is a small-molecule TKI that specifically targets growth factor receptors associated with angiogenesis and tumor cell proliferation. (VOTRIENT Prescribing Information. Research Triangle Park, NC: GlaxoSmithKline; 2010, Sloan B, Scheinfeld NS 2008) and has shown a significant response in treatment of advanced RCC in a study by Sternberg CN et al. [34].

Inlyta (Axitinib)

Approved by the FDA in January 2012, Axinitib is a prescription medicine used to treat advanced RCC when one prior drug treatment for this disease has not worked. In December 2011, the Oncologic Drugs Advisory Committee (ODAC) declared the recommendation of the approval of axitinib for the second-line treatment of patients with advanced renal cell carcinoma (RCC), based on the results of the Phase III trial comparing axitinib and Sorafenib.

Tivozanib (Aveo)

Aveo was approved in January 2012 and is an investigational TKI, designed to optimize blockade of the vascular endothelial growth factor (VEGF) pathway. In a Phase III trial of Aveo comparing with Sorafenib [TIVO-1 (Tivozanib Versus Sorafenib in 1st line Advanced

RCC)], Aveo demonstrated statistically significant progression-free survival (PFS) superiority versus an approved targeted agent (sorafenib) in advanced RCC [35].

Apart from TKI inhibitors, *Carfilzomib*, a novel proteasome inhibitor approved in 2009 demonstrated efficacy and was well tolerated in relapsed RCC *(http://www.asco.org/ascov2/Meetings/Abstracts?)*.

HIF Inhibitors

Hypoxia inducible factors (HIF) are transcription factors that play a very important role in oxygen sensing, delivering and adapting to oxygen deprivation in a cell. HiF-α, along with the constitutively expressed HiF-β subunit, bind to hypoxia-response elements in gene promoters to regulate the expression of genes that are involved in energy metabolism, angiogenesis, erythropoiesis, iron metabolism, cell proliferation, apoptosis and other biological processes [11].

HiF-1α and HiF-2α mediate transcription of a number of downstream genes thought to be important in cancer including transforming growth factor alpha (*TGFA*), platelet-derived growth factor (*PDGF*), and vascular endothelial growth factor (*VEGF*). HiF-2α was found to be more oncogenic in nature than HiF-1α, which activates pro-tumorigenic target genes [36].

Topotecan (Hycamtin)

Hycamtin is a chemotherapy agent that is also a topoisomerase I inhibitor. An *in-vitro* study of the effects of topotecan as a novel topoisomerase I inhibitor vs. 5 flouro-uracil (5-FU) in 20 RCC cell lines revealed that topotecan could effectively induce apoptosis in RCC cell lines than 5-FU at a clinical concentration of (< or = 1 microgm/ml) [37]. It is the water-soluble derivative of camptothecin and has also shown its effective use in many cancers such as lung, ovarian, cervical cancers including RCC [38].

Mammalian Target of Rapamycin (mTOR) Inhibitors

The mTOR signaling pathway was originally discovered during studies of the immunosuppressive agent rapamycin. This highly conserved pathway is known to regulate cell proliferation and metabolism in response to environmental factors, linking cell growth factor receptor signaling via phosphoinositide-3-kinase (PI-3K) to cell growth, proliferation, and angiogenesis. Loss of PTEN function through mutation, deletion, or epigenetic silencing results in increased activation of Akt and mTOR. The net effect is to stimulate cellular protein synthesis and entry of cells into the G1 phase of the cell cycle. Another product of this pathway is an increase in hypoxia inducible factor HiF-1α and HiF-2α expression, thus linking the mTOR pathway to angiogenesis.

The mammalian target of rapamycin (mTOR) also known as mechanistic target of rapamycin or FK506 binding protein 12-rapamycin associated protein 1 (FRAP1) is a protein which in humans is encoded by the *FRAP1* gene. mTOR is a serine/threonine protein kinase that regulates cell growth, cell proliferation, cell motility, cell survival, protein synthesis, and transcription. The mTOR pathway, which lies downstream of phosphatidylinositol-30 kinase, has also been a target for HIF in RCC.

Torisel (Temsirolimus)

Temsirolimus is a kidney cancer drug that was approved by FDA in late May 2007. It is a derivative of sirolimus and sold as Torisel. It was designed to inhibit the mTOR kinase, which is important in cell growth and cell survival. Temsirolimus is a specific inhibitor of mTOR and interferes with the synthesis of proteins that regulate proliferation, growth, and survival of tumor cells. Temsirolimus binds to an abundant intracellular protein, FKBP-12, and in this way forms a complex that inhibits mTOR signaling [39]. Treatment with temsirolimus leads to cell cycle arrest in the G1 phase, and also inhibits tumor angiogenesis by reducing synthesis of VEGF [40]. Temsirolimus has been shown to prolong survival, compared with interferon [41], in patients with previously untreated kidney cancer with high risk features in patients who have progressed while on sunitinib or sorafenib [42].

Afinitor (Everolimus or RAD001)

Everolimus, approved by the FDA in March 2009, is an orally administered mTOR inhibitor. Afinitor works by blocking mTOR and acts as a multifunctional inhibitor of cell growth and proliferation, angiogenesis, and cell metabolism. The drug is intended for use in patients with advanced renal cell cancer who have already tried a kinase inhibitor, such as Sutent or Nexavar. Everolimus has been associated with a modest prolongation of progression-free survival compared to placebo [42, 43]. This agent is definitely a reasonable second-line option in patients with advanced kidney cancer that have progressed on front-line therapy that targets the VEGF pathway [44, 45].

Conclusion

With advancement of science and technology, genitourinary cancers have become indispensible and subject to the vast array of basic and clinical research. The poor outcomes associated with metastatic RCC has driven the extensive studies for development of novel therapies, all thanks to the new era of translational medicine that have promised a new age of medicine 'From bench to bedside'. The identification of novel genes and their products and their investigative role in the pathogenesis of the disease will enable the development of several novel molecules that can help to increase the prognosis and overall survival of patients with metastatic RCC. Thus, the discovery of newer targeted molecules is an exciting field in the treatment of advanced renal cancers and clinical trials should be conducted to test these new agents for therapeutic implications of these approved agents.

Conflict of Interest

The authors declare no conflict of interest.

References

[1]   J.M Pow-Sang, *Cancer Control. 9*, 275, (2002).

[2]   L. Kopper and J. Timar, *Pathol Oncol Res. 12*, (2006).

[3]   R.J. Motzer, J. Bacik, L.H. Schwartz, V. Reuter, P. Russo, S. Marion, M. Mazumdar. *J Clin Oncol. 22*, 454, (2004).

[4]   B.J. Drucker. *Cancer Treat Rev. 31*, 536, (2005).

[5]   N.K. Vogelzang, W.M. Stadler. *Kidney Cancer. 352,* 1691, *(1997)*.

[6]   B. Curti, *JAMA. 292*, 97, (2004).

[7]   R.H. Weiss and P.Y. Li. *Kidney Int. 69*, 224, (2006)

[8]   M. Hurwitz, P.E. Spiess, J.A. Garcia, L.L. Pisters. Cancer Management, 14th Edition, Urothelial and Kidney Cancers, (2011).

[9]   D.F. McDermott, M.M. Regan M.B. Atkins. *Clin Genitourin Cancer. 5*, 114, (2006).

[10]   S.A. Rosenberg. *Nat Clin Pract Oncol. 4*, 497, (2007).

[11]   Therapies for Advanced Kidney Cancer, Kidney Cancer Association, *www.KidneyCancer.org*, Updated January 29th 2012.

[12]   S. Negrier, B. Escudier, C. Lasset, J.Y. Douillard, J. Savary, C. Chevreau, A. Ravaud, A. Mercatello, J. Peny, M. Mousseau, T. Philip, T. Tursz. *N Engl J Med. 338*, 1272, (1998).

[13]   C. Coppin, F. Porzsolt, A. Awa, J. Kumpf, A. Coldman, T. Wilt. *Cochrane Database Syst Rev. 25.*

[14]   CD001425 (2005). Review.

[15]   D.F. McDermott, M.M. Regan, J.I. Clark, L.E. Flaherty, G.R. Weiss, T.F. Logan, J.M. Kirkwood, M.S. Gordon, et al.. *J Clin Oncol. 23,* 133, (2005).

[16]   B. Escudier, C. Chevreau, C. Lasset, J.Y. Douillard, A. Ravaud, M. Fabbro, et al.. *J Clin Oncol.*,17 :2039, (1999).

[17]   S. Oudard, D. George, J. Medioni & R. Motzer. *Annals of Oncology. 18*, 25, (2007)

[18]   C. Pavlovich, L.S. Schmidt, J.L. Phillips. *Urol Clin North Am. 30*, 437,(2003).

[19]   F. Latif, K, Tory, J.R. Gnarra, M. Yao, F.M. Duh, M.L. Orcutt, T. Stackhouse, I. Kuzmin et al.. *Science. 260*, 1317, (1993).

[20]   J.R. Gnarra, K. Tory, Y. Weng, L. Schmidt, M.H. Wei, H. Li, F. Latif, S. Liu, F. Chen, F.M. Duh, et al.. *Nat Genet*, 7, 85 (1994).

[21]   S. Fleming. *Int J Dev Biol. 43*, 469, (1999).

[22]   W. Kim, W.G. Kaelin Jr. *Curr Opin Genet Dev. 13*, 55, (2003).

[23]   S.V. Ivanov, I. Kuzmin, M.H. Wei, S. Pack, L. Geil, B.E. Johnson, E.J. Stanbridge, M.I. Lerman. *Proc Natl Acad Sci U SA. 95*, 12596 (1998).

[24]   M. Ohh, R.L. Yauch, K.M. Lonergan, J.M.Whaley, A.O. Stemmer-Rachamimov, D.N. Louis et al.. *Mol Cell. 1*, 959, (1998).

[25]   A. Pause, S. Lee, R.A. Worrell, D.Y. Chen, W.H. Burgess, W.M. Linehan, R.D. Klausner. *Proc Natl Acad Sci USA. 94*, 2156, (1997).

[26]   P. Schraml, K. Struckmann, F. Hatz, S. Sonnet, C. Kully, T. Gasser, G. Sauter et al.. *J Pathol. 196,* 186, (2002).

[27]   M. Yao, M. Yoshida, T. Kishida, N. Nakaigawa, M. Baba, K. Kobayashi, T. Miura et al.. *J Natl Cancer Inst. 94*, 1569, (2002).

[28]   R.J. Motzer. *Crit Rev Oncol Hematol. 46*, Suppl: S 33. (2004). Review.

[29] J.C. Yang, L. Haworth, R.M. Sherry, P. Hwu, D.J. Schwartzentruber, S.L. Topalian, S.M. Steinberg, H.X. Chen, S.A. Rosenberg. *N Engl J Med. 31*, 427, (2003).

[30] B.I. Rini, S. Halabi, J. Taylor, E.J. Small, R.L. Schilsky; Cancer and Leukemia Group B. *Clin Cancer Res. 15*, 2584, (2004)

[31] C.A. Grandinetti, B.R. Goldspiel. *Pharmacotherapy. 27*, 1125, (2007)

[32] R.J. Motzer, T.E. Hutson, P. Tomczak, M.D. Michaelson, R.M. Bukowski, O. Rixe, S.Oudard, S. Negrier, C. Szczylik, S.T. Kim, I. Chen, P.W. Bycott, C.M. Baum, R.A. Figlin. *N Engl J Med. 356*, 115, (2007).

[33] S. Radulovic, S.K. Bjelogrlic. *J BUON. 12,* Suppl 1:S151, (2007).

[34] B. Drucker, J. Bacik, M. Ginsberg, S. Marion, P. Russo, M. Mazumdar, R. Motzer. *Invest New Drugs. 21*, 341, (2003).

[35] C.N. Sternberg. *Clin Adv Hematol Oncol. 8*, 232, (2010).

[36] R. Motzer et al.. ASCO Annual Meeting, Abstract Number 4501, (2012).

[37] M.M. Baldewijns, I.J. van Vlodrop, P.B. Vermeulen, P.M. Soetekouw, M. van Engeland, A.P. de Bruïne. *J Pathol. 221*, 125, (2010). Review.

[38] U. Ramp, C. Mahotka, T. Kalinski, E. Ebel, H.E. Gabbert, C.D. Gerharz. *Anticancer Res. 21*, 3509, (2001).

[39] A. Rapisarda, J. Zalek, M. Hollingshead, T. Braunschweig, B. Uranchimeg, C.A. Bonomi, S.D. Borgel, J.P. Carter, S.M. Hewitt, R.H. Shoemaker, G. Melillo. *Cancer Res. 64*, 6845, (2004).

[40] M.W. Harding. *Clin Cancer Res. 9*, 2882, (2003). Review.

[41] X. Wan, N. Shen, A. Mendoza, C. Khanna, L.J. Helman. *Neoplasia. 8*, 394, (2006).

[42] G.R. Hudes. *Clin Adv Hematol Oncol. 5*, 772, (2007).

[43] G.R. Hudes. *Cancer. 15* (10 Suppl), 2313, (2009). Review.

[44] R.J. Motzer, B. Escudier, S. Oudard, T.E. Hutson, C. Porta, S. Bracarda, V. Grünwald, J.A. Thompson, R.A. Figlin, N. Hollaender, G. Urbanowitz, W.J. Berg, A. Kay, D. Lebwohl, A. Ravaud; RECORD-1 Study Group. *Lancet. 9*, 449, Epub (2008).

[45] W. M Linehan, G Bratslavsky, P.A. Pinto, L.S.Schmidt, L. Neckers, D. Bottaro, and R. Srinivasan. *Annu Rev Med. 61,* 329, (2010).

[46] S.S. Agarwala, S. Case. *Oncologist. 15*, 236, Epub (2010).

In: Handbook of Genitourinary Medicine: New Research   ISBN: 978-1-62618-226-4
Editor: Rashmi R. Singh   © 2013 Nova Science Publishers, Inc.

Chapter II

Matrix Metalloproteinases: Role in Urothelial Cancer

Rama Devi Mittal and Priyanka Srivastava

Department of Urology and Renal Transplantation,
Sanjay Gandhi Post Graduate Institute of Medical Science,
Raebareli Road, Lucknow, Uttar Pradesh, India

Abstract

Metastatic spread of cancer continues to be the greatest barrier to cancer cure. Hence, matrix metalloproteinases (MMPs) have been implicated in metastases in understanding the strategy to contest the disease. MMPs contribute to the carcinogenic process at multiple stages. Thus, the most promising and exciting applications of MMPs in human cancers is as potential cancer biomarkers, both diagnostic and prognostic that can be exploited as tools for early detection, disease progression, and metastasis of urological cancers.

Markers associated with the progression of bladder carcinoma (BC) are well established. However, paucity of definitive clinical prognostic markers and targets still remain. Search for molecular targets that may predict which superficial bladder tumors will later progress to become invasive is required. Appropriate molecular targets that regulate BC metastasis are an important step in identifying and creating newer generation chemotherapeutics with improved efficacy and fewer side effect profiles. Over-expression of the matrix metalloproteinases MMP-2 and MMP-9 offers prognostic value as markers of disease-specific survival. These molecules have been implicated in metastasis of BC, but the underlying mechanisms through which they are controlled are poorly defined. Majority of the biomarkers studied in patients with BC have focused on urine. Studies have shown that urinary MMP-2 and MMP-9 levels correlate with presence of BC as well as stage and grade of disease. Increased levels of MMP-9 and MMP-2 in urine correlate with increased expression of these proteases in bladder tumor tissue as well.

MMP-2, -9, -15, and -26 expressions in tissue or serum have been positively correlated with Gleason score in prostate cancer (PCa). Among these MMPs, the activities of plasma MMP-2 and -9 increased significantly in metastatic PCa. Analysis of

MMP-2 and -9 levels in radical prostatectomy specimens revealed these two as significant predictors of cancer recurrence. These two enzymes may also be markers of therapeutic efficacy, since both the levels and activities of plasma MMP-2 and -9 decreased significantly in metastatic patients after therapy. In addition, increased urinary MMP-9 activity has been shown to distinguish between prostate and other types of cancer (e.g., BC).

All these strategies may lead to breakthroughs for preventive interventions in the field of the molecular epidemiology of urological cancers.

Introduction

One of the most hazardous public health problems known to date is cancer. Several million deaths from cancer are registered every year worldwide. Intensive development of modern preventative measures against cancer is being developed every year, since prevention of a disease is much easier than its treatment. Diagnostic tests and targeted therapy are the common modes of treatment. However, in-spite of novel improvements in screening and prevention modalities, the prognosis of patients in urological cancer, remains poor. Thus, the aim of modern molecular biology and medicine is to develop adequate novel genomic markers with predictive, therapeutic, and prognostic significance. Some of these markers may evaluate the predisposition to disease as well as reveal risk groups in populations, and thereafter, a complex of preventive measures among risk-group subjects may be conducted.

One of the most important genomic markers is the single nucleotide polymorphism (SNP), which represents a variation in DNA sequence, when a single nucleotide differs between members of a biological species or paired chromosomes in an individual. The presence of such a substitution in DNA sequence may often cause a deviation of protein function and/or lead to disruption of exonic splicing enhancer sequences. SNP's may lead to changes in transcription factors and vary the efficiency of gene expression, as well as introduce an alternative translation initiation codon that may lead to down regulation of the wild-type transcript. Hence, SNP's can be very informative and are extensively used in studies of their association with risk for many cancers. Therefore, it is feasible to say that identification of SNPs as markers of cancer predisposition are a convenient, simple, and effective way to identify and treat various malignancies in the earliest stages.

Metastatic spread of cancer continues to be the greatest barrier to cancer cure. Understanding the molecular mechanisms of metastasis is crucial for the design and effective use of novel therapeutic strategies to combat metastases. One class of molecules that has been repeatedly implicated in metastasis is the matrix metalloproteinases (MMPs). MMPs are a multigene family of zinc-dependent endopeptidases that share a similar structure and which collectively, have the capacity to degrade virtually every component of the extracellular matrix (ECM). Expression of various MMPs has been reported to up regulate virtually every type of human cancer and correlates with advanced stage, invasive and metastatic properties and, in general, poor prognosis. Both MMP-2 and MMP-9 have been implicated in the induction of the angiogenic switch in different model systems. Further, up-regulation of MMP expression, in particular, the gelatinases, can degrade basement membrane components, allows the tumor cells to invade into the adjacent stroma and to break down the basement membranes associated with capillaries and lymphatic vessels allowing tumor cells to enter the circulation. Remotely MMPs are required for local migration, establishment of a microenvironment conducive for metastatic growth, and angiogenesis for sustained growth. Thus, MMPs contribute to the carcinogenic process at multiple stages. One of the more promising and exciting applications of MMPs in human cancers is as potential cancer biomarkers, both diagnostic and prognostic, that can be exploited as tools for early detection, disease progression, and metastasis of urological cancers.

While most MMPs promote tumor progression, some of them may protect the host against tumorigenesis in a context-dependent manner. MMPs have been chosen as promising targets for cancer therapy on the basis of their aberrant up-regulation in malignant tumors and their ability to promote cancer metastasis [1, 2]. This broad range of activity has led to considerable interest in the use of MMPs in the clinical setting as diagnostic or prognostic biomarkers and as therapeutic targets.

Metastasis and Matrix Metalloproteinase

Human cells are surrounded by collagen fibers and connective tissue. In order to grow and expand, healthy cells need to break down this extra-cellular barrier that confines them. This process is essential for life and for this reason; cells produce and secrete various enzymes that digest connective tissue components, including collagen and elastin. It is important that these enzymes, called matrix metalloproteinases or MMPs, be regulated by sets of activators and inhibitors so that the integrity of the connective tissue is never compromised.

Tumor metastasis is a multistep process by which a subset or individual cancer cells disseminate from a primary tumor to distant secondary organs or tissues. Tumor cells fulfill their metastatic potential after acquiring those advantageous characteristics, which allow them to escape from the primary tumor, migrate and invade surrounding tissues, enter the vasculature, circulate and reach secondary sites, extravasate, and establish metastatic foci [1, 3, 4, 5]. All these steps of the metastatic cascade require from tumor cells some survival and communication skills. Failure to overcome challenges imposed by normal physiological barriers often leads to tumor cell death or clearance, thereby making each phase of metastasis apparently a rate-limiting step [2, 6]. The ability of cancer cells to migrate from the tissue of origin and metastasize to surrounding or distant organs is essential for tumor progression. Many studies of tumor invasion and metastases have focused on the degradation of the extracellular matrix and endothelial cell basement membrane by MMPs.

Matrix Metalloproteinases and Cancer

Excessive disintegration of connective tissue accompanies pathology and once this disintegration occurs, infectious cancer cell microbes (including viruses) can invade tissues. In extreme cases, such as in cancer, the excessive production of digestive enzymes and the disintegration of collagen and connective tissue by cancer cells are the dangerous mechanisms by which these cells invade and spread to other organs. MMPs have biological characteristics that allow them to target multiple cells and act on various levels of these inflammatory and destructive processes (Figure 1). Thus, it is crucial to understand the temporal expression and individual contribution of each MMP in the initiation and progression of BC to allow for development of a selective and specific target. Past experiences have shown that a broad spectrum MMP inhibitor could be of limited benefit. What the consequences of MMP inhibition are on the protective immunity and tissue repair should be a concern to be investigated because these enzymes have natural biological functions related to various substrates and numerous tissues.

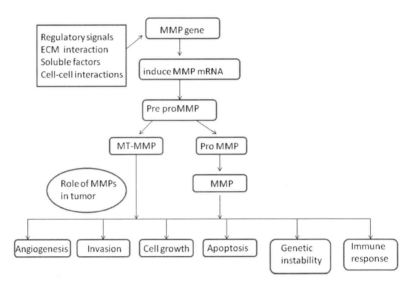

Figure 1. Proposed flow chart to demonstrate how the MMPs involved in the pathways can affect the susceptibility to cancer (self drawn).

Bladder Cancer

Carcinogenesis of human Bladder cancer (BC) is a multistep process, and metastasis represents a critical step in carcinogenesis. Markers associated with the progression of bladder carcinoma, such as depth of invasion, stage, grade, and multiplicity are well established. Paucity of definitive clinical prognostic markers and targets still remain. Therefore, there is a need to identify those molecular targets that may predict which superficial bladder tumors will later progress to become invasive. Appropriate molecular targets that regulate BC metastasis are an important step in identifying and creating newer generation chemotherapeutics with improved efficacy and fewer side effect profiles. Extensive work on the mechanism of tumor invasion and metastasis has identified MMPs as the key players in tumor spread. In transitional cell carcinoma (TCC), the most common form of BC, overexpression of the matrix metalloproteinases MMP-2 and MMP-9 offers prognostic value as markers of disease-specific survival. These molecules have been implicated in metastasis of BC, but the underlying mechanisms through which they are controlled are poorly defined. Majority of the biomarker studies in patients with BC have focused on urine. Studies have shown that urinary MMP-2 and MMP-9 levels correlate with presence of BC as well as stage and grade of disease. Increased levels of MMP-9 and MMP-2 in urine correlate with increased expression of these proteases in bladder tumor tissue as well.

Prostate Cancer

The importance of the bone microenvironment to the pathophysiology and morbidity associated with prostate cancer (PCa) bone metastasis is becoming increasingly apparent. Significant alterations take place in the microenvironment of bone, which disturb the normal coupling that exists between bone resorption and bone formation. Consequently, a better understanding of the mechanisms that interact at the molecular level will definitely result in more effective therapy for patients with this devastating complication of prostatic carcinoma.

MMP-2, -9, -15, and -26 expressions in tissue or serum have been positively correlated with Gleason score (A Gleason score is given to PCa based upon its microscopic appearance. Cancers with a higher Gleason score are more aggressive and have a worse prognosis) in PCa. Among these MMPs, the activities of plasma MMP-2 and -9 increased significantly in metastatic PCa. Analysis of MMP-2 and -9 levels in radical prostatectomy specimens revealed these two as significant predictors of cancer recurrence. These two enzymes may also be markers of therapeutic efficacy, since both the levels and activities of plasma MMP-2 and -9 decreased significantly in metastatic patients after therapy. In addition, increased urinary MMP-9 activity has been shown to distinguish between prostate and other types of cancer (e.g., BC). All these strategies may lead to breakthroughs for preventive interventions in the field of the molecular epidemiology of cancer.

Urothelial Cancers

Urothelial carcinomas show a divergent biological behavior, which significantly complicates risk stratification and clinical management. The recent shift to an agnostic genome-wide association approach led to the identification of several cancer susceptibility loci, and provided valuable leads for new mechanistic insights into urothelial carcinogenesis. The markers do not have sufficient discriminatory ability yet to be applied for risk assessment in the population and the question is whether they ever will. Prognostic and predictive studies in cancer are still in their infancy compared with etiologic studies.

However, it is increasingly clear that genetic factors also play an important role in determining BC risk [3, 7]. Although many genetic factors are involved in the development of BC, interactions between neoplastic cells and the surrounding microenvironment are crucial for tumorigenesis. The MMP activity regulates the functionality of multiple extracellular matrix proteins, cytokines, growth factors and cell signaling and adhesion receptors. Aberrantly enhanced MMP proteolysis affects multiple cell functions, including proliferation, migration and invasion [4, 8].

Matrix Metalloproteinases and Urothelial Cancers

PCa is most common disease of developed countries, however, in India, its incidence is quite low which may be due to difference in ethnicity, lifestyle and most importantly left undiagnosed, due to lack of awareness and established structural screening program However, the incidence is likely to increase owing to changing lifestyle and increasing health awareness in India. The genetic basis leading to PCa and its progression is poorly understood. MMPs are responsible for cancer invasion and metastasis. Increased plasma/serum levels of certain MMPs have been reported in patients with cancer. MMP-2, -9, -15, and -26 expressions in tissue or serum have been positively correlated with Gleason score in PCa [9, 11]. Our data indicated that MMP2-1306C/T gene polymorphism contributes to PCa susceptibility. These findings suggested MMP2 variants as a predictor of PCa progression risk among North Indian men [12]. Among these MMPs, the activities of plasma MMP-2 and -9 increased significantly in metastatic PCa [13]. Furthermore, over expression of MMP-2 in cancer tissue was associated with shorter disease-free survival in a study with T3N0-2M0 patients [14]. Analysis of MMP-2 and -9 levels in radical prostatectomy specimens revealed these two as significant predictors of cancer recurrence [15]. These two enzymes may also be markers of therapeutic efficacy, since both the levels and activities of plasma MMP-2 and -9 decreased significantly in metastatic patients after therapy [13]. In addition, increased urinary MMP-9 activity has been shown to distinguish between prostate and other types of cancer (e.g., BC) [16]. MMPs can also be combined with other markers to increase their predictive capability. For example, the mRNA ratio of gelatinases (MMP-2 and MMP-9) to E-cadherin in biopsy samples independently predicted (PCa) stage [17]. A disintegrin and metalloprotease (ADAM8) levels in PCa tissue has been significantly correlated with higher tumor status, positive nodal status, and higher Gleason scores [18]. Higher ADAM9 levels were associated with shortened prostate-specific antigen relapse-free survival [19].

As is expected, a majority of the biomarker studies in patients with BC have focused on urine and blood. Studies from our group have shown that MMP-1 and MMP-2, MMP-3, MMP-7 and MMP-9 correlate with presence of BC as well as stage and grade of disease [20-22]. Roy et al. reported the identification of several MMP species in urine from patients with primary tumors in the bladder and prostate including MMP-2, MMP-9, MMP-9 neutrophil gelatinase-associated lipocalin complex and MMP-9 dimer [16]. Each urinary MMP species was detected at significantly higher rates in urine from patients with cancer as compared with controls. The difference in detection of MMP species in the urine of the two types of cancers studied may serve as a tumor-specific fingerprint that can indicate both the presence of a tumor as well as its location [16]. Increased levels of MMP-9 and MMP-2 in urine correlate with increased expression of these proteases in bladder tumor tissue as well [23]. Urinary MMP-9 levels when combined with telomerase analysis of exfoliated cells from voided urine could also increase the sensitivity of cytology, a commonly used method for BC detection and monitoring [24]. ADAM12 mRNA and protein were found to be upregulated in BC tissue and urinary ADAM12 levels were higher in patients with BC [25].

Genome Wide Association Studies (GWAS) of MMPs

The relatively new genome-wide association study approach has investigated hundreds of thousands of genetic variants across the whole human genome for association with cancer. Results from GWAS have shown that cancer risks associated with common variation are very low and large studies are required to confirm associations [26]. This suggests that conflicting results for previous numerous candidate gene studies were at least partly due to paucity of power to detect such low risks. All GWAS in cancer done to date, surprisingly SNPs located within the MMP gene family have not been identified. Whereas, it is acknowledged that virtually all GWAS designs to date have been underpowered to detect the effect sizes that were subsequently confirmed by replication studies [27], and thus many cancer-associated SNPs remain to be identified. Another possible explanation could be poor coverage of MMP genes by current methodologies. The coverage of MMP SNPs by the Hap- Map database has been reported to be as low as 30% [28], which may partly explain their failure to be identified by published GWAS. Also, by definition, the SNPs included in GWAS designs have a minimum frequency of 5%, and thus risk-associated SNPs occurring at lower frequencies would not be detected using current scans. Moreover, considering the role of MMPs in the degradation of the ECM, it is possible that these genes are likely to be involved in cancer progression. Hence, MMP SNPs may be more strongly associated with prognosis rather than predisposition. However, current published GWAS have not directly examined associations of SNPs with cancer progression, and investigation of surrogates of prognosis such as grade have been limited by relatively poor availability of detailed clinical information from the cohorts studied. These studies suggest that despite the emergence of GWAS, there is still a need for the identification of MMP candidate gene studies of cancer predisposition and role in prognosis of disease.

Genetic Polymorphisms in Matrix Metalloproteinase Genes and Relevance to Cancer Care

Certain polymorphisms alone, in combination or by interaction with environmental factors may affect the angiogenic pathway and thereby susceptibility and/or severity of cancers. Detection of the role of angiogenic gene polymorphisms that influence cancer susceptibility and/or severity may improve our understanding of tumors angiogenesis and may influence risk stratification and detection, use of new treatment strategies and prognostication of disease. In addition to regulating the growth of primary and secondary tumors, MMPs promote tumors angiogenesis and metastasis by ECM remodeling. Altered MMP expression occurs in tumors of the oesophagus, stomach, colorectal, pancreatic, breast, prostate, lung and ovary with levels correlating with disease stage and possibly. In our previous case-control study analysis was done to see the frequency distribution as well as association of MMP gene polymorphism like *MMP1 (-519) A/G, MMP1 (-1607) A/G, MMP3(-1612 A/G), MMP3 (+5356A/G), MMP3 (+1161G/A), MMP3 (-1171 5A/6A), MMP7 (-181 A/G) F, MMP9 (381 C/G), MMP9 (836) Q279R A/G, MMP9(P574R)G/C* and *MMP9(R668Q)G/A* in controls and patients with susceptibility to BC.

MMP1 SNPs and Its Relevance to Cancer

MMPs are essential for tumor cells to penetrate the basement membrane and colonize distant sites. Among MMPs, *MMP1* is the most ubiquitously expressed interstitial collagenase, thereby claiming a prominent role in collagen degradation [29]. Clinical research showed the presence of *MMP1* in cancer cells, and that *MMP1* expression is associated with a poor prognosis [30].

Our study revealed that*MMP1* 519 was not associated with BC risk or with any confounding factors. The frequency distribution of *MMP1 (-519 A/G)* in controls was AA 52.5%, AG 37.5% and GG 10.0% (Figure 2). In the other polymorphic site of *MMP1* 1607, it is assumed that the insertion of a guanine nucleotide in the 2G allele of the *MMP1* 1607 1G/2G polymorphism, may create a core binding site for transcription factor Ets, leading to a significantly higher promoter activity [31]. This polymorphism has also been associated with susceptibility to diverse diseases (Table 1). This feature indicated that patients carrying the 2G allele may be predisposed to the development of cancers and/or their rapid progression [32-37]. The 2G allele in polymorphism −1607 of *MMP1* may potentially increase the level of protein expression. This mechanism may provide the molecular basis for a more intense degradation of ECM, which is important in tissue remodeling and repair during development and inflammation.

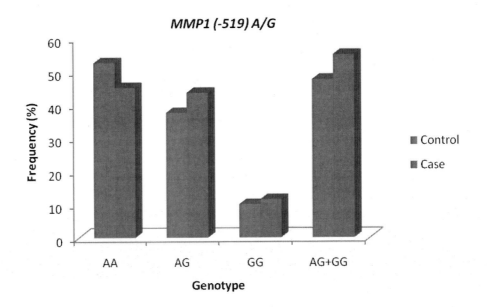

Figure 2. MMP1 (-519) A/G gene polymorphism in Bladder cancer patients.

MMP1 SNPs have been correlated with the risk of BC in Caucasian population [38], renal cell carcinoma in Japanese population [39] and colorectal cancer in Caucasian population [40]. Our study showed that the frequency of the 2G allele was significantly higher in BC patients compared to the controls (p = 0.002; OR 2.29), suggesting that variations in the *MMP1* promoter could affect BC initiation and development (Figure 3).

Our results were compatible to the study of Tasci et al.., 2008, who reported *MMP1* 2G allele to be significantly associated with the risk of BC in Turkish population [33]. Hirata et al.., (2003) reported that the frequency of the 2G/2G genotype was significantly higher in patients with RCC than in controls [39]. Zhu et al.., 2001 also showed that there was a significant association between the 2G/2G genotype and lung cancer risk [41].

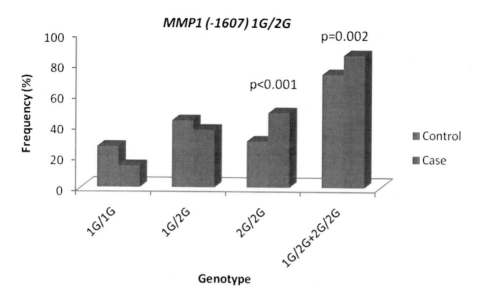

Figure 3. MMP1 (-1607) 1G/2G gene polymorphism in Bladder cancer patients.

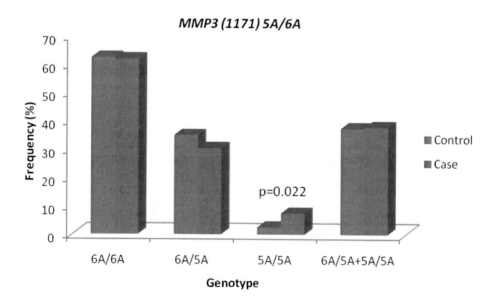

Figure 4. MMP3 (1171) 5A/6A gene polymorphism in Bladder cancer patients.

However, some representative studies demonstrated conflicting results, since this SNP generally displays ethnic variations. To determine whether a true difference exists between the genotype distributions in different races, Ju et al.., (2007) compared the genotype distribution of the *MMP1 –1607* SNP in different populations from Korea, Japan, Taiwan, USA, UK, France, Italy, Poland and Brazil [56]. The results showed that the allele frequencies of *MMP1–1607* SNP in Asians showed no significant difference, but significant variation in allele frequencies were observed in white populations [56], indicating ethnic variation between Asians and Caucasians.

Table 1. Polymorphisms in the *MMP1* gene associated with some diseases

MMP1 -1607 1G/2G			
Disease	Population	Population number of test group/control group	Reference
Bladder cancer	North India	200/200	Present study
Ovarian cancer	Japan	163	[30]
Lung cancer	Caucasian	456/451	[41]
Renal cell carcinoma	Japan	156/230	[39]
Sclerosing cholangitis	Norway	165/346	[42]
Colorectal cancer	France	201	[40]
Glioblastoma	USA	81/57	[43]
Oral carcinoma	China	96/120	[44]
Prostate cancer	Turky	55/43	[45]
Bladder cancer	Caucasian	242 /312 Invasive/superficial	[38]
Colorectal cancer	Korean	185/304	[34]
Brain astrocytoma	China	221/266	[46]
Peripheral arterial occlusive	Italy	157/206	[47]
Oral carcinoma	Japan	170/164	[48]
Oral cancer	Greece & Germany	156/141	[49]
Nasopharyngeal carcinoma	Tunisia	174/171	[50]
Bladder cancer	Turky	102/94	[33]
Implant failure	Brazil	55/60	[51]
Severe chronic periodontitis	Turky	102/98	[52]
Degenerative disc disease	Southern China	378/122	[53]
Endobronchial tuberculosis	Taiwan	38 of 101 pulmonary TB	[54]
Prostate cancer	Japan	283/251	[55]
Oral submucous fibrosis	India	412/426	[35]
Head & Neck squamous cell carcinoma	India	422/426	[35]
Glioblastoma Multiforme	North India	110/150	[36]
Lung cancer	China	825/825	[37]

MMP3 SNPs and Its Relevance to Cancer

MMP3 has the potential to degrade a wide range of extracellular matrix proteins and activates some other members of the MMP family, making it likely a key player in extracellular matrix degradation and remodeling. A single adenine insertion/deletion polymorphism (5A/6A) at the -1171 position of the *MMP3* promoter region causes elevation of the transcriptional level and local expression of *MMP3* [57, 58]. The polymorphism is due to variation in the length of a polymonomeric track of adenosines located relative to the transcription start site, resulting in one allele having five adenosines (5A) and the other allele having six adenosines (6A).

Okamoto et al.., (2010) suggested *MMP3* 5A allele to be perhaps a cooperative risk factor for poor prognosis in hepatocellular carcinoma (HCC) patients [59]. Ye et al.., (1996) in their study opined 5A allele to have a greater promoter activity as compared to 6A allele in fibroblasts and vascular smooth muscle [57]. The influence of this SNP in the *MMP3* promoter on development and invasiveness of tumors was not consistent in different tumor types. In our study, individuals with *MMP3-1171 (5A/5A)* genotype were at higher risk of BC (Figure 4), whereas in study by other investigators in colorectal cancer higher risk was associated with 6A/6A genotype, in a Japanese cohort [60]. An Italian study in breast cancer demonstrated association of 5A allele with susceptibility and suggested an unfavorable prognostic feature associated with more invasive disease [61]. A study by Choudhary et al.., (2010) concluded that the expression of *MMP3* genotype associated with the 5A alleles may have an important role in the susceptibility of the patients to develop Oral Submucous Fibrosis (OSMF) and Head and Neck Squamous Cell Carcinoma (HNSCC [35]) . The two other SNPs, rs520540 and rs679620, also did not modulate susceptibility to BC in our population (Figure 5, 6), as well as in study by Shibata et al.., (2005) in Alzheimer's disease [62].

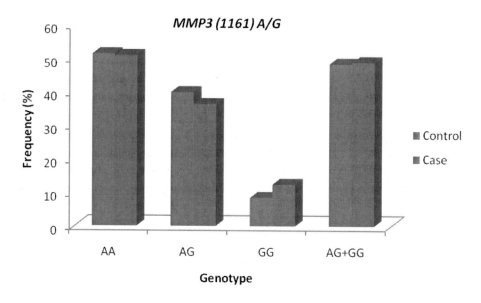

Figure 5. MMP3 (1161) A/G gene polymorphism in Bladder cancer patients.

MMP7 SNPs and Its Relevance to Cancer

Two polymorphisms exist in the *MMP7* promoter region, −181A/G and −153 C/T which are known to modify the gene transcription activity [64, 65]. Numerous studies have shown association of *MMP7 −181A/G* polymorphisms with malignant diseases [66-70]. However, till date, association of the *MMP7* functional polymorphism −181A/G with risk of BC has not been demonstrated. Wu et al.., (2006) reported that *MMP7* is highly expressed in metastatic cervical squamous cell carcinoma, and may serve as a marker in estimating the invasive and metastatic potential of cervical squamous cell carcinoma [71]. Yi et al.., (2010) suggested that individuals with the *MMP7 -181* G/G and A/G genotype may have an increased risk of developing endometrial cancer [72].

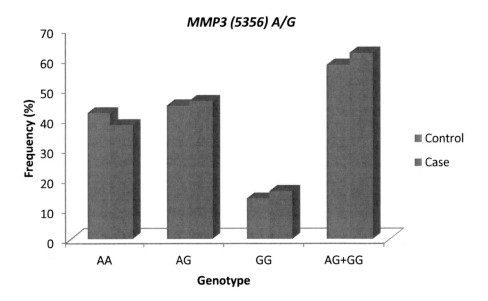

Figure 6. MMP3 (5356) A/G gene polymorphism in Bladder cancer patients.

Table 2. Polymorphisms in the *MMP3-1171 5A/5A* gene associated with some cancers

MMP3-1171 5A/5A			
Disease	Population	Population number of test group/control group	Reference
Bladder cancer	North India	200/200	Present study
Colorectal cancer	Japan	102/94	[60]
Breast cancer	Italy	156/230	[61]
Alzheimer's disease	Japan	--	[62]
Esophageal adenocarcinoma	Canada	313/455	[63]
Oral Submucous Fibrosis	India	101/126	[35]
Head and Neck Squamous Cell Carcinoma	India	135/126	[35]
Hepatocellular carcinoma	Japan	92 patients	[59]

Our results showed that individuals with *MMP7* 181GG genotypes and 181G allele were at significant increased risk of BC (p=0.005; OR=2.38) (Figure 7). Another study in North India by Achyut et al.., (2009) revealed significant association of functional *MMP-7* gene variants toward susceptibility to H. pylori-induced precancerous gastric lesions [73] Malik et al.., (2011) suggested that *MMP7 (181A>G)* genetic polymorphism may contribute to squamous cell gastric cancer susceptibility and also reported that GG carriers are at a higher risk of esophageal squamous cell carcinoma in the Kashmir valley [36]. Wu et al.., (2011) reported that *MMP7* G allele carriers were at significantly higher risk of cervical cancer [74]. The underlying mechanism for this association may be related to the promoter activity variation of the 181G alleles. It is assumed that functional analysis of *MMP7* 181G alleles could increase the gene transcription activity as suggested by Jormsj"o etal (2001) [65]. A study by Saarialho-Kere et al.., (1995) has found that presence of 181G variant allele resulted in a higher level of *MMP7* expression [75]. Presence of high expression *MMP7* 181G allele may alter cell surface signaling including cellular proliferation, invasion and apoptosis processes [76]. Therefore, individuals with excess *MMP7* activity by harboring the 181G allele may be predisposed to malignant transformation. In addition, enhanced expression of *MMP7* due to 181G allele may lead to increased activation of other members of the MMP family such as *MMP2*. Association of *MMP7* 181G allele with gastric ulcer, colorectal carcinoma, and ovarian cancer risk has also been reported [66, 69, and 77].

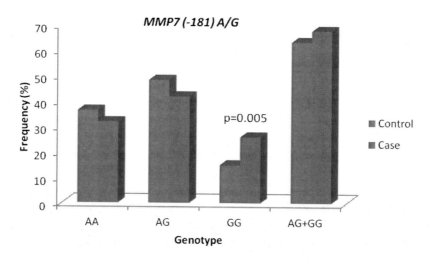

Figure 7. MMP7 (-181) A/G gene polymorphism in Bladder cancer patients.

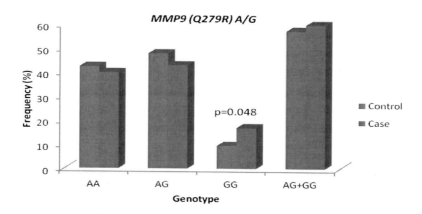

Figure 8. MMP9 (Q279R) A/G gene polymorphism in Bladder cancer patients.

Table 3. Polymorphisms in the *MMP7* gene associated with some cancers

MMP7 (-181 A/G)			
Disease	Population	Population number of test group/control group	Reference
Bladder cancer	North India	200/200	Present study
Colorectal carcinoma	Italy	58/111	[66]
Gastric cardiac carcinoma	China	201/350	[77]
Gastric ulcer	Germany	599 patients	[67]
Ovarian cancer	North China	---	[69]
Cervical squamous cell carcinoma	China	86/21	[71]
Oral cancer	Greece	159/120	[78]
Cervical cancer	North India	150/162	[79]
Hepatocellular carcinoma	China	434/480	[80]
Gastric precancerous lesions	North India	130/200	[73]
Endometrial cancer	Taiwan	118/229	[72]
Esophageal squamous cell carcinoma	Kashmir	135/195	[36]
Gastric cancer	Kashmir	108/195	[36]
Cervical cancer	China	--	[74]

MMP9 SNPs and its Relevance to Cancer

MMP9 plays an important role in several cancers, including BC [81]. The main function of *MMP9* is in degradation of type IV collagen, a major component of the basement membrane, which is breached in invasive BC. Matsumura et al.., (2005) reported that genotypes containing -1562T allele was associated with increased risk of gastric cancer [82]. In addition, Hu et al.., (2005) showed that the nonsynonymous SNP P574R may predicate risk of development and metastasis of lung cancer [83]. Our study demonstrated that the Q279R, P574R polymorphism of *MMP9* was associated with increased risk of BC (Figures 8, 9). Furthermore, the results indicated that individuals carrying 279R-574R and 279Q-574R haplotypes could be predisposed to occurrence of BC. These data clearly demonstrated that the *MMP9* polymorphism is a putative risk factor of BC in Indian population. *MMP9* gene variants have also been associated with risk for metastasis in lung cancer, in-transit metastasis in melanoma cancer, and higher grade in renal cell carcinoma [83-85]. In a study by Tang et al.., (2008) significant association was found between the two nonsynonymous *MMP9* polymorphisms and lymph node metastasis in gastric cancer [86]. Similar results were found by Hu et al.., (2005) in lung cancer [83]. Jin et al.., (2009), in their study observed *MMP9* Arg279Gln and Arg668Gln SNPs to be potential predictors of survival in (Non-small cell lung carcinoma) NSCLC patients [87]. Study of Wu et al.., (2008) shows that *MMP9* gene P574R polymorphism may contribute to a genetic risk factor for esophageal squamous cell carcinoma in Chinese population [88]. Fang et al.., (2010) reported that *MMP9 279R/Q* alleles and genotypes may be associated with the risk of colorectal carcinoma in Han Chinese [89]. In a recent study by Casabonne et al.., (2011), *MMP9* gene was found to be at highest risk of chronic lymphocytic leukemia [90]. Screening of SNP rs3025079, rs3918248 did not show the polymorphism, compatible with a Japanese study [62].

Table 6.4. Polymorphisms in the *MMP9* gene associated with some cancers

MMP9			
Disease	Population	Population number of test group/control group	Reference
Bladder cancer	North India	200/200	Present study
Gastric cancer	Japan	177/224	[82]
Lung cancer	China	744/747	[83]
Alzheimer's disease	Japan	--	[62]
Renal cell carcinoma	Japan	179/211	[85]
Cutaneous Malignant Melanoma	USA	1002 patients	[84]
Esophageal squamous cell carcinoma	China	---	[88]
Gastric cancer	China	74/100	[86]
Non-small cell lung cancer	China	561 patients	[87]
Cervical cancer	USA	101/273	[91]
Colorectal carcinoma	China	237/252	[89]
Chronic lymphocytic leukemia	Europe	240/515	[90]

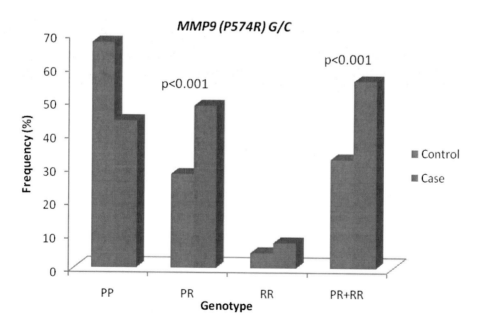

Figure 9. MMP9 (P574R) G/C gene polymorphism in Bladder cancer patients.

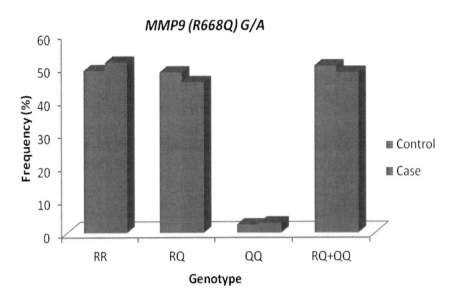

Figure 10. MMP9 (R668Q) G/A gene polymorphism in Bladder cancer patients.

Conclusion

Mesenchymal/stromal cell interactions in health and disease involve MMPs and involve multiple ligands and cellular signaling pathways. The variations in the levels of MMPs between the epithelium and the stroma, their cross talk, and associated interactions are likely to be critically important in the development of a number of urological disorders such as cancer. Useful markers associated with molecular aggressiveness might be of vital in predicting the conclusion of malignancies and to better recognize patient groups that need more aggressive treatment. Furthermore, the introduction of novel prognostic markers might promote exclusively new treatment possibilities and there is an undeniable need of markers that could be used as novel therapies, as the existing therapies have made no difference in survival of these patients in the last 50 years. Further research is required for the development of their potential diagnostic and therapeutic possibilities.

The data regarding influences of MMP genotypes on susceptibility to and progression of cancer discussed above are pertinent to the understanding of the genetic basis and biological mechanisms underlying the pathogenesis of these complex diseases. These genetic data support the notion that MMPs play important roles in the development of these diseases which all involve extracellular matrix remodelling.

References

[1]   K. Pantel, R.H. Brakenhoff, *Nat. Rev. Cancer, 4*, 448 (2004).
[2]   H. Hua, M. Li, T. Luo, Y. Yin, Y. Jiang, *Cell Mol. Life Sci. 68*, 3853 (2011).
[3]   D. Hanahan, R.A. Weinberg, *Cell, 144*, 646 (2011).
[4]   A.F. Chambers, A.C. Groom, I.C. MacDonald, *Nat. Rev. Cancer, 2*, 563 (2002).

[5]   D.H. Geho, R.W. Bandle, T. Clair, L.A Liotta, *Physiology (Bethesda), 20*, 194 (2005).

[6]   R.O. Hynes, *Cell, 113*, 821 (2003).

[7]   X. Wu, H. Zhao, R. Suk, D.C. Christiani, *Oncogene, 23*, 6500 (2004).

[8]   A.V. Chernov, A.Y. Strongin, *Biomol Concepts, 2*, 135 (2011).

[9]   M. Wood, K. Fudge, J.L. Mohler, A.R. Frost, F. Garcia, M. Wang, M.E. Stearns, *Clin. Exp. Metastasis, 15*, 246 (1997).

[10]   C.G. Sauer, A. Kappeler, M. Späth, J.J. Kaden, M.S. Michel, D. Mayer, U. Bleyl, R. Grobholz, *Virchows Arch. 444*, 518 (2004).

[11]   A.C. Riddick, C.J. Shukla, C.J. Pennington, R. Bass, R.K. Nuttall, A. Hogan, K.K. Sethia, V. Ellis, A.T. Collins, N.J. Maitland, R.Y. Ball, D.R. Edwards, *Br J Cancer, 92*, 2171 (2005).

[12]   P. Srivastava, T.A. Lone, R. Kapoor, R.D. Mittal, *Arch Med Res. 43*, 117 (2012).

[13]   G. Morgia, M. Falsaperla, G. Malaponte, M. Madonia, M. Indelicato, S. Travali, M.C. Mazzarino, *Urol Res. 33*, 44 (2005).

[14]   D. Trudel, Y. Fradet, F. Meyer, F. Harel, B. Têtu, *Hum Pathol. 39*, 731 (2008).

[15]   H. Miyake, M. Muramaki, T. Kurahashi, A. Takenaka, M. Fujisawa, *Urol Oncol. 28*, 145 (2010).

[16]   R. Roy, G. Louis, K.R. Loughlin, D. Wiederschain, S.M. Kilroy, C.C. Lamb, D. Zurakowski, M.A. Moses, *Clin Cancer Res. 14*, 6610 (2008).

[17]   H. Kuniyasu, R. Ukai, D. Johnston, P. Troncoso, I.J. Fidler, C.A. Pettaway, *Clin Cancer Res. 9*, 2185 (2003).

[18]   F.R. Fritzsche, M. Jung, C. Xu, A. Rabien, H. Schicktanz, C. Stephan, M. Dietel, K. Jung, G. Kristiansen, *Virchows Arch. 449*, 628 (2006).

[19]   F.R. Fritzsche, M. Jung, A. Tölle, P. Wild, A. Hartmann, K. Wassermann, A. Rabien, M. Lein, M. Dietel, C. Pilarsky, D. Calvano, R. Grützmann, K. Jung, G. Kristiansen, *Eur Urol. 54*, 1097 (2008).

[20]   P. Srivastava, R. Gangwar, R. Kapoor, R.D. Mittal, *Dis Markers, 29*, 37 (2010a)

[21]   P. Srivastava, A. Mandhani, R. Kapoor, R.D. Mittal, *Ann Surg Oncol. 17*, 3068 (2010b).

[22]   P. Srivastava, R. Kapoor, R.D. Mittal , *Urol Oncol.* (2011) [Epub ahead of print]

[23]   A.S. Papathoma, C. Petraki, A. Grigorakis, H. Papakonstantinou, V. Karavana, S. Stefanakis, F. Sotsiou, A. Pintzas,. *Anticancer Res. 20*, 2009 (2000).

[24]   S. Eissa, M. Swellam, H. el-Mosallamy, M.S. Mourad, N. Hamdy, K. Kamel, A.S. Zaglol, M.M. Khafagy, O. el-Ahmady, *Anticancer Res. 23*, 4347 (2003).

[25]   C. Fröhlich, R. Albrechtsen, L. Dyrskjøt, L. Rudkjaer, T.F. Ørntoft, U.M. Wewer, *Clin Cancer Res. 12*, 7359 (2006).

[26]   F. Kronenberg, *Exp. Gerontol. 43*, 39 (2008).

[27]   D. Altshuler, M. Daly, *Nat Genet. 39*, 813 (2007).

[28]   E. Tantoso, Y. Yang, K.B. Li, *BMC Genomics, 7*, 238 (2006).

[29]   W.G. Stetler-Stevenson, L.A. Liotta, D.E. Jr. Kleiner, *FASEB J. 7*, 1434 (1993).

[30]   Y. Kanamori, M. Matsushima, T. Minaguchi, K. Kobayashi, S. Sagae, R. Kudo, N. Terakawa, Y. Nakamura, *Cancer Res. 59*, 4225 (1999).

[31]   S. Ye, P. Eriksson, A. Hamsten, M. Kurkinen, S.E. Humphries, A.M. Henney, *J Biol Chem. 271*, 13055 (1996).

[32] R. Nishizawa, M. Nagata, A.A. Noman, N. Kitamura, H. Fujita, H. Hoshina, T. Kubota, M. Itagaki, S. Shingaki, M. Ohnishi, H. Kurita, K. Katsura, C. Saito, H. Yoshie, R. Takagi, *BMC Cancer*, 7, 187 (2007).

[33] A.I. Tasci, V. Tugcu, E. Ozbek, B. Ozbay, A. Simsek, V. Koksal, *BJU Int. 101*, 503 (2008).

[34] M. Woo, K. Park, J. Nam, J.C. Kim, *J Gastroenterol Hepatol.* 22, 1064 (2007).

[35] A.K. Chaudhary, M. Singh, A.C. Bharti, M. Singh, S. Shukla, A.K. Singh, R. Mehrotra, *BMC Cancer, 10*, 369 (2010).

[36] N. Malik, R. Kumar, K.N. Prasad, P. Kawal, A. Srivastava, A.K. Mahapatra, *J Neurooncol. 102*, 347 (2011).

[37] L. Liu, J. Wu, C. Wu, Y. Wang, R. Zhong, X. Zhang, W. Tan, S. Nie, X. Miao, D. Lin, *Cancer*, (2011). doi: 10.1002/cncr.26154. (Epub ahead of print)

[38] A.K. Kader, J. Liu, L. Shao, C.P. Dinney, J. Lin, Y. Wang, J. Gu, H.B. Grossman, X. Wu, *Clin Cancer Res. 13*, 2614 (2007).

[39] H. Hirata, K. Naito, S. Yoshihiro, H. Matsuyama, Y. Suehiro, Y. Hinoda, *Int J Cancer, 106*, 372 (2003).

[40] F. Zinzindohoué, T. Lecomte, J.M. Ferraz, A.M. Houllier, P.H. Cugnenc, A. Berger, H. Blons, P. Laurent-Puig, *Clin Cancer Res. 11*, 594 (2005).

[41] Y. Zhu, M.R. Spitz, L. Lei, G.B. Mills, X. Wu, *Cancer Res. 61*, 7825 (2001).

[42] K. Wiencke, A.S. Louka, A. Spurkland, M. Vatn, E. Schrumpf, K.M. Boberg; IBSEN Study Group, *J Hepatol. 41*, 209 (2004).

[43] J. McCready, W.C. Broaddus, V. Sykes, H.L. Fillmore, *Int J Cancer, 117*, 781 (2005).

[44] Z.G. Cao, C.Z. Li, *Oral Oncol. 42*, 32 (2006).

[45] S. Albayrak, O. Cangüven, C. Göktaş, H. Aydemir, V. Köksal, *Urol Int. 79*, 312 (2007).

[46] Z. Lu, Y. Cao, Y. Wang, Q. Zhang, X. Zhang, S. Wang, Y. Li, H. Xie, B. Jiao, J. Zhang, *J Neurooncol. 85*, 65 (2007).

[47] A. Flex, E. Gaetani, F. Angelini, A. Sabusco, C. Chillà, G. Straface, F. Biscetti, P. Pola, J.J. Jr Castellot, R. Pola, *J Intern Med. 262*, 124 (2007).

[48] R. Nishizawa, M. Nagata, A.A. Noman, N. Kitamura, H. Fujita, H. Hoshina, T. Kubota, M. Itagaki, S. Shingaki, M. Ohnishi, H. Kurita, K. Katsura, C. Saito, H. Yoshie, R. Takagi, *BMC Cancer*, 7, 187 (2007).

[49] E. Vairaktaris, C. Yapijakis, S. Derka, Z. Serefoglou, S. Vassiliou, E. Nkenke, V. Ragos, A. Vylliotis, S. Spyridonidou, C. Tsigris, A. Yannopoulos, C. Tesseromatis, F.W. Neukam, E. Patsouris, *Anticancer Res. 27*, 459 (2007).

[50] H.B. Nasr, S. Mestiri, K. Chahed, N. Bouaouina, S. Gabbouj, M. Jalbout, L. Chouchane, *Clin Chim Acta. 384*, 57 (2007).

[51] M.F. Leite, M.C. Santos, A.P. de Souza, S.R. Line, *Int J Oral Maxillofac Implants, 23*, 653 (2008).

[52] D. Pirhan, G. Atilla, G. Emingil, T. Sorsa, T. Tervahartiala, A. Berdeli, *J Clin Periodontol. 35*, 862 (2008).

[53] Y.Q. Song, D.W. Ho, J. Karppinen, P.Y. Kao, B.J. Fan, K.D. Luk, S.P. Yip, J.C. Leong, K.S. Cheah, P. Sham, D. Chan, K.M. Cheung, *BMC Med Genet. 9*, 38 (2008).

[54] H.P. Kuo, Y.M. Wang, C.H. Wang, C.C. He, S.M. Lin, H.C. Lin, C.Y. Liu, K.H. Huang, L.L. Hsieh, C.D. Huang, *Tuberculosis (Edinb), 88*, 262 (2008).

[55] N. Tsuchiya, S. Narita, T. Kumazawa, T. Inoue, Z. Ma, H. Tsuruta, M. Saito, Y. Horikawa, T. Yuasa, S. Satoh, O. Ogawa, T. Habuchi, *Oncol Rep. 22*, 493 (2009).

[56] W. Ju, J.W. Kim, N.H. Park, Y.S. Song, S.C. Kim, S.B. Kang, H.P. Lee, *J Obstet Gynaecol Res. 33*, 155 (2007).

[57] S. Ye, P. Eriksson, A. Hamsten, M. Kurkinen, S.E. Humphries, A.M. Henney, *J Biol Chem. 271*, 13055 (1996).

[58] S. Ye, G.F. Watts, S. Mandalia, S.E. Humphries, A.M. Henney, *Br Heart J. 73*, 209 (1995).

[59] K. Okamoto, C. Ishida, Y. Ikebuchi, M. Mandai, K. Mimura, Y. Murawaki, I. Yuasa, *Intern Med. 49*, 887 (2010).

[60] Y. Hinoda, N. Okayama, N. Takano, K. Fujimura, Y. Suehiro, Y. Hamanaka, S. Hazama, Y. Kitamura, N. Kamatani, M. Oka, *Int J Cancer, 102*, 526 (2002).

[61] G. Ghilardi, M.L. Biondi, M. Caputo, S. Leviti, M. DeMonti, E. Guagnellini, R.Scorza, *Clin Cancer Res. 8*, 3820 (2002).

[62] N. Shibata, T. Ohnuma, S. Higashi, C. Usui, T. Ohkubo, A. Kitajima, A. Ueki, M. Nagao, H. Arai, *Neurobiol Aging, 26*, 1011 (2005).

[63] P.A. Bradbury, R. Zhai, J. Hopkins, M.H. Kulke, R.S. Heist, S. Singh, W. Zhou, C. Ma, W. Xu, K. Asomaning, M. Ter-Minassian, Z. Wang, L. Su, D.C. Christiani, G. Liu, *Carcinogenesis, 30*, 793 (2009).

[64] L.E. Jones, M.J. Humphreys, F. Campbell, J.P. Neoptolemos, M.T. Boyd, *Clin Cancer Res. 10*, 2832 (2004).

[65] S. Jormsjö, C. Whatling, D.H. Walter, A.M. Zeiher, A. Hamsten, P. Eriksson, *Arterioscler Thromb Vasc Biol. 21*, 1834 (2001).

[66] G. Ghilardi, M.L. Biondi, M. Erario, E. Guagnellini, R. Scorza, *Clin Chem. 49*, 1940 (2003).

[67] S. Hellmig, S. Ott, P. Rosenstiel, U.F. Robert, J. Hampe, S. Schreiber, *Am J Gastroenterol, 101*, 29 (2006).

[68] J. Zhang, X. Jin, S. Fang, R. Wang, Y. Li, N. Wang, W. Guo, Y. Wang, D. Wen, L. Wei, Z. Dong, G. Kuang, *Carcinogenesis, 26*, 1748 (2005).

[69] Y. Li, X. Jin, S. Kang, Y. Wang, H. Du, J. Zhang, W. Guo, N. Wang, S. Fang, *Gynecol Oncol. 101*, 92 (2006).

[70] E. Vairaktaris, Z. Serefoglou, C. Yapijakis, A. Vylliotis, E. Nkenke, S. Derka, S. Vassiliou, D. Avgoustidis, F.W. Neukam, E. Patsouris, *Anticancer Res. 27*, 2493 (2007).

[71] S.H. Wu, J. Zhang, Y. Li, J.M. Li, *Ai Zheng, 25*, 315 (2006).

[72] Y.C. Yi, P.T. Chou, L.Y. Chen, W.H. Kuo, E.S. Ho, C.P. Han, S.F. Yang, *Clin Chem Lab Med. 48*, 337 (2010).

[73] B.R. Achyut, U.C. Ghoshal, N. Moorchung, B. Mittal, *DNA Cell Biol. 28*, 295 (2009).

[74] S. Wu, S. Lu, H. Tao, L. Zhang, W. Lin, H. Shang, J. Xie, *J Huazhong Univ Sci Technolog Med Sci. 31*, 114 (2011).

[75] U.K. Saarialho-Kere, E.C. Crouch, W.C. Parks, *J Invest Dermatol. 105*, 190 (1995).

[76] C. Yu, K. Pan, D. Xing, G. Liang, W. Tan, L. Zhang, D. Lin, *Cancer Res. 62*, 6430 (2002).

[77] J. Zhang, X. Jin, S. Fang, R. Wang, Y. Li, N. Wang, W. Guo, Y. Wang, D. Wen, L. Wei, Z. Dong, G. Kuang, *Carcinogenesis, 26*, 1748 (2005).

[78] E. Vairaktaris, C. Yapijakis, S. Derka, Z. Serefoglou, S. Vassiliou, E. Nkenke, V. Ragos, A. Vylliotis, S. Spyridonidou, C. Tsigris, A. Yannopoulos, C. Tesseromatis, F.W. Neukam, E. Patsouris, *Anticancer Res. 27*, 459 (2007).

[79] H. Singh, M. Jain, B. Mittal, *Gynecol Oncol. 110*, 71 (2008).

[80] W. Qiu, G. Zhou, Y. Zhai, X. Zhang, W. Xie, H. Zhang, H. Yang, L. Zhi, X. Yuan, X. Zhang, F. He, *Cancer Epidemiol Biomarkers Prev. 17*, 2514 (2008).

[81] Y. St-Pierre, C. Van Themsche, P.O. *Curr Drug Targets Inflamm Allergy, 2*, 206 (2003).

[82] S. Matsumura, N. Oue, H. Nakayama, Y. Kitadai, K. Yoshida, Y. Yamaguchi, K. Imai, K. Nakachi, K. Matsusaki, K. Chayama, W. Yasui, *J Cancer Res Clin Oncol. 131*, 19 (2005).

[83] Z. Hu, X. Huo, D. Lu, J. Qian, J. Zhou, Y. Chen, L. Xu, H. Ma, J. Zhu, Q. Wei, H. Shen, *Clin Cancer Res. 11*, 5433 (2005).

[84] J. Cotignola, B. Reva, N. Mitra, N. Ishill, S. Chuai, A. Patel, S. Shah, G. Vanderbeek, D. Coit, K. Busam, A. Halpern, A. Houghton, C. Sander, M. Berwick, I. Orlow, *BMC Med Genet. 8*, 10 (2007).

[85] Y. Awakura, N. Ito, E. Nakamura, T. Takahashi, H. Kotani, Y. Mikami, T. Manabe, T. Kamoto, T. Habuchi, O. Ogawa, *Cancer Lett. 241*, 59 (2006).

[86] Y. Tang, J. Zhu, L. Chen, L. Chen, S. Zhang, J. Lin, *Clin Cancer Res. 14*, 2870 (2008).

[87] G. Jin, R. Miao, Z. Hu, L. Xu, X. Huang, Y. Chen, T. Tian, Q. Wei, P. Boffetta, H. Shen, *Int J Cancer, 124*, 2172 (2009).

[88] J. Wu, L. Zhang, H. Luo, Z. Zhu, C. Zhang, Y. Hou, *DNA Cell Biol. 27*, 553 (2008).

[89] W.L. Fang, W.B. Liang, H. He, Y. Zhu, S.L. Li, L.B. Gao, L. Zhang, *DNA Cell Biol. 29*, 657 (2010).

[90] D. Casabonne, O. Reina, Y. Benavente, N. Becker, M. Maynadié, L. Foretová, P. Cocco, A. González-Neira, A. Nieters, P. Boffetta, J.M. Middeldorp, S. de Sanjose, *Haematologica, 96*, 323 (2011).

[91] R. Brooks, N. Kizer, L. Nguyen, A. Jaishuen, K. Wanat, E. Nugent, P. Grigsby, J.E. Allsworth, J.S. Rader, *Gynecol Oncol. 116*, 539 (2010).

In: Handbook of Genitourinary Medicine: New Research   ISBN: 978-1-62618-226-4
Editor: Rashmi R. Singh   © 2013 Nova Science Publishers, Inc.

Chapter III

Toll-like Receptor Genes and Prostate Cancer Risk

Rama Devi Mittal and Raju Kumar Mandal

Department of Urology and Renal Transplantation,
Sanjay Gandhi Post Graduate Institute of Medical Science,
Uttar Pradesh, India

Abstract

Prostate cancer is one of the most common non-cutaneous malignant neoplasms and a major cause of morbidity and mortality in men in many industrialized countries. Several determinants such as age, ethnicity, family history along with genetic susceptibility and Inflammation have been implicated in prostate cancer. Causes of inflammation are diverse, including infectious diseases, stress and environmental exposure. Chronic inflammation can incite carcinogenesis by enhancing the secretion of growth factors such as cytokines, chemokines and inducing oxidative stress by the release of nitric oxide (NO) and reactive oxygen species (ROS). These somatic modifications may be responsible for the progression from chronic inflammation of the prostate (prostatitis) to prostate carcinogenesis. Many pathogens have been detected in the prostate, suggesting the role of bacterial and viral sequences in the activation of Toll-like receptors (TLRs) that might positively or negatively influence tumorigenesis by triggering the innate and adaptive immune responses.

TLRs constitute a family of receptors and play a pivotal role in immune responses that directly recognize antigen determinants of viruses, bacteria, protozoa, and fungi. Hence, they play a key role in the activation of the adaptive immune response to eliminate infectious pathogens and cancer debris. TLRs that recognize lipid and protein ligands (TLR1, TLR2, TLR4, TLR5 and TLR6) are expressed on the plasma membrane, whereas TLRs that detect viral nucleic acids (TLR3, TLR7, and TLR9) are localized in lysosomal compartments.

Polymorphisms that directly influence TLR expression may thus be implicated in a skewed/unregulated inflammatory response to infection, rendering the host more susceptible to prostate carcinogenesis. Sequence variants in several TLR genes have been linked to prostate cancer risk, such as TLR4 and the TLR6-TLR1-TLR10 gene cluster;

TLRs mediate the enhanced immune responses induced by many immuno-adjuvants, suggesting that increased TLR activation may stimulate anticancer immunity. Thus, enhanced TLR activity could inhibit carcinogenesis while decreased activity could allow cancer cells to escape immune detection and elimination. Alternatively, TLR activation may promote carcinogenesis by creating a pro-inflammatory environment that enhances tumor growth and chemo-resistance and/or result in chronic inflammation-induced immune suppression that allows cancer progression. Further basic and clinical research into the effects of TLR activation will be essential before making accurate predictions of how variation in TLR action will influence cancer risk.

Introduction

Prostate cancer is the most common non-cutaneous malignancy in men in Western countries, accounting for one-third of all male cancer diagnoses and 9% of all deaths due to cancer. The number of afflicted men is increasing rapidly as the population of males over the age of 50 grows worldwide. Prostate cancer is a heterogeneous disease with multiple loci contributing to its susceptibility; therefore, finding strategies for the prevention of prostate cancer is a crucial medical challenge. Surgery, radiation, and chemotherapy are the most common options for localized prostate cancer treatment; however, recurrence or metastasis eventually lead to death for ~30,000 patients every year [1]. Because the average life expectancy is continuously rising, it is estimated that there will be a 2.5-fold increase in the incidence of prostate cancer by the year 2050 [2]. While several determinants such as age, ethnicity, and family history have been implicated in prostate cancer aetiology, other risk factors remain elusive. It is well established that genetic factors also play a significant role in pathogenesis of prostate cancer [3].

Possible Cause of Inflammation in Prostate Cancer

Approximately 20% of all human cancers in adults result from chronic inflammatory states and chronic inflammation, which are triggered by infectious agents or exposure to other environmental factors, or by a combination there of. Clinical and epidemiological studies have suggested a strong association between chronic infection, inflammation, and cancer. Inflammation seems to play a role in carcinogenesis by causing cellular and genomic damage, promoting cellular turnover, and creating a tissue microenvironment that can enhance cell replication, angiogenesis and tissue repair [4]. Actually, tumours are thought to develop from chronic Inflammation, where uncontrolled cell proliferation occurs in a milieu rich in pro-inflammatory cytokines, inflammatory mediators, and growth factors normally involved in chronic and unresolved inflammation [5]. In normal tissues, anti-inflammatory cytokines are synchronically upregulated after the pro-inflammatory cytokines are produced, leading to inflammation resolution. In chronic inflammation, this does not occur, resulting in a continuous production of reactive oxygen species, leading to oxidative DNA damage and reduced DNA repair, and increased proliferation [5]. It is known that there are two main prostate pathologies affecting men during their lifetime: benign prostatic hypertrophy (BPH) and prostate cancer. In most cases, the cause of prostatic inflammation is unclear. Various potential sources exist for the initial inciting event, including direct infection, urine reflux inducing chemical and physical trauma, dietary factors, oestrogens, or a combination of two or more of these factors (Fig. 1). Furthermore, any of these could lead to a break in immune tolerance and the development of an autoimmune reaction to the prostate.

Areas of inflammation are extremely common in the prostate, with studies reporting a prevalence of >95% in resection specimens particularly involving the peripheral zone of the prostate where prostate cancer typically occurs [6, 7]. Many different pathogenic organisms have been observed to infect and induce an inflammatory response in the prostate. These include sexually transmitted organisms, such as Neisseria gonorrhoeae, Chlamydia trachomatis, Trichomonas vaginalis and Treponema pallidum, and non-sexually transmitted bacteria such as Propionibacterium acnes and those known to cause acute and chronic bacterial prostatitis, primarily Gram-negative organisms such as Escherichia coli [8]. Recently a gamma xenotropic meurine leukemia related virus (XMRV) was detected in prostate cancer specimen using DNA microarrays based analysis [9]. The virus was detected primarily in men with a specific germline mutation of RNASEL, the gene that encodes for the antiviral enzyme RNASEL, suggesting that prolonged infection in the prostate may be a result of genetic predisposition. Although each of these pathogens has been identified in the prostate, the extent to which they typically infect this organ varies.

Sexually transmitted diseases (STDs) are hypothesized to play a role in the development of prostate cancer, frequent sexual encounters with prostitutes and unprotected sexual intercourses were shown to be associated with increased risk of STDs, such as syphilis and gonorrhoea resulted in severe prostatic inflammation or prostatic abscess and associated with an increased risk for prostate cancer [10, 11]. A meta-analysis showed an increased prostate cancer risk directly associated with the number of sexual partners and history of sexually transmitted infection. Taylor et al.. 2005 also demonstrated significantly increased risk for prostate cancer in subjects affected by gonorrhoea and HPV infection [12]. Other indicators of promiscuous sexual behaviour and of exposure to STDs, including number of sexual partners, age at first intercourse, and frequency of sex, have each been reported to be associated with prostate cancer risk in previous studies [13]. Viruses such as Human papillomavirus (HPV), cytomegalovirus (CMV), human herpes simplex virus type 2 (HSV2) and human herpes virus type 8 (HHV8) have been detected in the prostate [14, 15]. Prolonged infection could trigger an inflammatory reaction that persists despite clearance of the organism by the unmasking of the self antigens in an autoimmune manner. In support of this, T cells responses against histone peptides and prostate specific antigen (PSA) have been detected in the prostate. How frequently these agents infect the prostate, and whether they elicit an inflammatory response, is largely unknown and it is still unknown if there is a role of the different pathogens that can infect the prostate in the development of prostate cancer.

Role of PIA in Prostate Cancer Development

The human prostate gland is a common site of inflammation; histologically most lesions that contain either acute or chronic inflammatory infiltrates in the prostate are associated with atrophic epithelium or focal epithelial atrophy. Atrophy of the prostate is identified as a reduction in the volume of pre existing glands and stroma and can be divided into two major patterns, diffuse and focal. Diffuse atrophy results from a decrease in circulating androgens and involves the entire prostate in a relatively uniform manner. In contrast, focal atrophy is not related to decrease circulating androgens, and it occurs as patches of atrophic epithelium within a background of surrounding normal-appearing nonatrophic epithelium [16]. They are also located mainly in the prostatic peripheral zone. Repeated injury to the prostate epithelium by oxidative or nitrosamine damage from inflammatory cells, in response to pathogens or autoimmune disease from direct injury from circulating carcinogens and toxins derived from the diet or from urine reflux to the prostate, causes morphological change called proliferative inflammatory atrophy (PIA). The association between PIA and chronic inflammation suggests that the lesions, caused by regenerative proliferation of the epithelial cells in response to injury caused by inflammatory oxidants and the hyperproliferative state, may lead to cancer. They have demonstrated transition between areas of PIA with Prostatic intraepithelial neoplasia (PIN) [17]. High-grade PIN is frequently observed in proximity to PIA, and morphologic transitions between high-grade PIN and PIA frequently occur within the same acinus/duct [18]. In a recent European study by Tomas et al.. 2007; analyzing different types of atrophy in normal of benign hyperplastic prostatic tissue and in prostate cancer tissue, they found an association between PIA and prostate cancer. PIA was significantly more frequent in prostates with carcinoma (1.63 vs 1.27 atrophic lesions per slide) (p=0.001), whereas Proliferative Atrophy (PA) displayed an increased frequency in BPH (2.28 vs 0.76 atrophic lesions per slide) (p=0.001) [19].

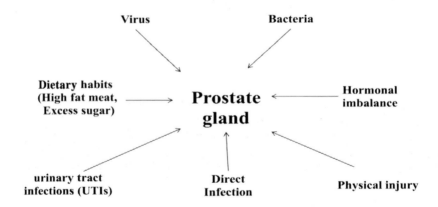

Figure 1. Possible causes of prostatic inflammation.

Toll-like Receptors (TLRs): A Possible Link between inflammation and Prostate Cancer

Challenge by Invading pathogens has led multicellular organisms to develop a number of defensive measures for the recognition and clearance of infectious agents. The innate immune (non-specific) system is the first lines of defence against invading microorganisms, which manifest as inflammation, are crucial for the initiation of adaptive (specific) immune responses. Therefore, the seemingly divergent effects of inflammation and immuno-editing are paradoxical. The normal prostate populated by a small number of T cells, B lymphocytes, macrophages and mast cells, and T lymphocytes can be seen as early as 12 weeks of gestation [20]. However, most adult prostate tissues contain increased inflammatory infiltrates, although the extent and type of inflammation are variable.

Toll-like receptors (TLRs) is a type 1 transmembrane protein with an extracellular domain play a pivotal role in immune responses, being involved in the regulation of inflammatory reactions and activation of the adaptive immune response to eliminate infectious pathogens and cancer debris. TLRs comprise a family of germ line encoded membrane bound receptors which recognize conserved bacterial, viral, fungal and protozoan molecular structures in the extracellular compartment. They are called pathogen associated molecular patterns (PAMPs). Of them most prominent is lipopolysaccharide (LPS) from gram negative bacteria. To date, in mammals, the 'TLR family' consists of 11 members. They are a special form of pattern recognition receptors (PRRs) that can recognize specific classes PAMP in different microorganisms (Table 1). Most TLRs are transmembrane proteins with a large extracellular domain and an intracellular TIR (Toll/IL-1 receptor) domain. One of the major signal transduction pathways of TLRs is mediated through an adaptor protein, MyD88, which can bind to TIR domain and further recruit down-stream signalling proteins ultimately leading to activation of transcriptional factors, such as NF-kB (a nuclear factor of kappa light polypeptide gene enhancer in B-cells) and AP-1, resulting in the expression of genes cytokines, interleukin related to inflammatory responses (Fig 2). Recognition of PAMPs by TLR-expressing cells result in acute responses necessary to clear the pathogens in host. High levels of proinflammatory cytokines were found in prostatic tissue samples and in semen of patients with chronic prostatitis [21], as well as in prostatic fluid collected from prostatectomy [22]. Members of the TLR family are expressed in different amounts in various types of cells and expression of all TLRs on the transcriptomic or proteomic level was detected in prostate [23].

Table 1. TLRs and their respective chromosome and PAMPs

TLR	Chromosome	PAMP	Microorganism
TLR1	4p14	TLR2 cofactor	Bacteria
TLR2	4q31-32	Lipopolysaccharide, lipoteichoic acid, peptidoglycan, Zymosan	Bacteria, viruses and fungi
TLR3	4q35	dsRNA	Viruses
TLR4	9q32-33	Lipopolysaccharide, Heat-shock protein 60/70-Host	Gram negative bacteria and Viruses
TLR5	1q41-42	Flagellin	Gram-positive and Gram-negative bacteria
TLR6	4p14	Peptidoglycan	Gram-positive and Gram-negative bacteria
TLR7	Xp22	Single-strand RNA	virus
TLR8	Xp22	Single-strand RNA	virus
TLR9	3p21	CpG-containing DNA	Bacteria and virus
TLR10	4p14	Prokaryotic DNA	Bacteria

Single nucleotide polymorphisms (SNPs) may result in amino acid substitutions altering protein function or splicing; they can change the structure of enhancer sequences during splicing or affect mRNA stability. SNPs may alter transcription factor binding motifs, changing the efficacy of enhancer or repressor elements, and can also alter the structure of translation initiation codons that may lead to the down regulation of the wild type transcript [24].

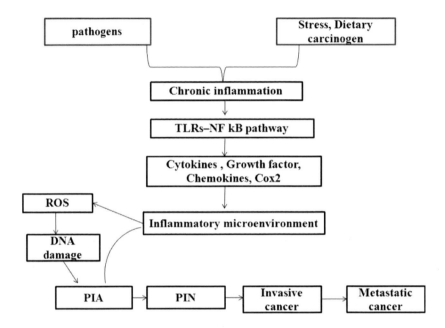

Figure 2. Chronic Inflammation produced by pathogen (Bacteria, Virus) and Stress, Dietary carcinogen activate the TLR-NF-kB pathway. These transcription factors coordinate the production of inflammatory cytokine, growth factors and chemokines, which activate the key transcription factors in inflammatory cell and tumor cells, resulting more cancer related inflammatory microenvironment being generated. Which lead to release ROS, ROS can interact with DNA in the proliferating epithelial prostate cell to produce permanent mutation.

Taking into account the key role of TLRs in prostate cancer development and immune tumor evasion, sequence variations of these genes have been identified and implicated in susceptibility of many cancers including prostate cancer [25]. Therefore, polymorphisms in TLR genes of the inflammatory pathway could influence disease susceptibility and progression by altering the response to infection and downstream inflammatory effects. We performed a study to evaluate the influence of TLR2 (-196 to -174 Del), TLR3 (c.1377C/T) and TLR9 (G2848A) genes polymorphism in prostate cancer from North India [26]. Our cohort included 195 prostate cancer patients and 250 controls. Genotyping was carried out from blood DNA, using PCR RFLP methodology. The del/del genotype inclined to be more frequent among patients than control subjects (3.1% vs. 2.0%, p= 0.309). The variant allele (D) carrier (ID + DD) was higher in cases (30.8%) than in control (22.8%), the result showed statistically significant risk (p= 0.040; OR= 1.57) with prostate cancer. The TLR3 and 9 genotypic and allelic frequency distributions between cases and healthy controls were similar demonstrating no association for the risk of prostate cancer (Fig 3-5). Our result did not observe any significant association with any tumor grade. Further, we also performed case only analysis with smoking status with these polymorphisms and observed no significant association.

Previous studies has demonstrated that TLRs, specifically TLR subclass 4 (TLR4) and TLR9, may contribute to prostate cancer pathogenesis by stimulating prostate epithelial cell proliferation in response to infectious stimuli [27]. SNPs that directly manipulate TLR expression may thus be implicated in a skewed/unregulated inflammatory response to infection, rendering the host more susceptible to prostate carcinogenesis.

Table 1. Genetic Variants of TLRs investigated for prostate cancer risk

Genetic variants	Population	Results	Reference
TLR1			
rs5743551	Sweden	Increased risk	[28]
rs5743556	Sweden	Increased risk	[28]
rs5743604	Sweden	Increased risk	[28]
rs5743611	Sweden	Increased risk	[28]
rs4624663	Sweden	Increased risk	[28]
rs4833095	USA	Reduced risk	[29]
rs5743596	USA	Reduced risk	[29]
rs5743551	USA	Reduced risk	[29]
TLR2			
rs3804100	Sweden	No association	[30]
TLR3			
rs3775296	Sweden	No association	[30]
rs5743305	Sweden	No association	[30]
rs5743313	Sweden	No association	[30]
TLR4			
rs11536889	Korean	Increased risk	[31]
rs1927911	Korean	Increased risk	[31]
rs11536858	Korean	No Association	[31]
rs1927914	Korean	No association	[31]
rs11536891	Korean	No association	[31]
rs11536897	Korean	No association	[31]

To date vast number of TLR polymorphisms have been identified, and the functional implications of the majority of these variations are unknown [25]. Despite there being some fundamental mechanisms that indicate TLR gene polymorphisms may play a role in prostate cancer aetiology, and despite there being a number of comprehensive studies conducted on large samples in various countries and results have also varied slightly in different populations. However, it is possible that some of the TLR gene polymorphisms may be the markers of prostate cancer risk in certain populations (Table 2), most studies have done within TLR4 and the TLR6-TLR1-TLR10 gene cluster located within a 54 kb region on chromosome 4p14. Several variant alleles within the TLR4 gene are reported to be associated with prostate cancer risk, suggesting a role of TLR4 genetic variant in prostate cancer risk. Significant associations were also reported for variant alleles within the TLR6-TLR1-TLR10 gene cluster, and similarly to TLR4, inverse significant associations were observed.

Inconsistent association results are a major concern for disease association studies and often reflect heterogeneity of study design and composition, as well as emphasizing the complex nature of genetic contributions to a multifaceted disease such as prostate cancer.

Table 2. Genetic Variants of TLRs investigated for prostate cancer risk

Genetic variants	Population	Results	Reference
TLR5			
rs1053954	Sweden	No association	[30]
rs2072493	Sweden	No association	[30]
rs5744113	Sweden	No association	[30]
rs5744174	Sweden	No association	[30]
TLR6			
rs5743788	USA	No association	[32]
rs5743795	USA	No association	[32]
rs5743806	USA	No association	[32]
rs5743810	Taiwan	No association	[32]
TLR7			
rs179008	Sweden	No association	[30]
rs179019	Sweden	No association	[30]
Rs2302267	Sweden	No association	[30]
TLR8			
rs1548731	Sweden	No association	[30]
rs4830806	Sweden	No association	[30]
rs5744068	Sweden	No association	[30]
TLR9			
rs187084	Sweden	No association	[30]
TLR10			
rs11096955	USA	Reduced risk	[29]
rs11096957	USA	Reduced risk	[29]
rs4129009	Sweden	Reduced risk	[28]

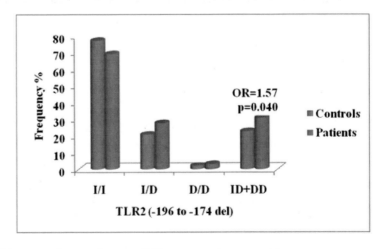

Figure 3. TLR2 gene variants and susceptibility to prostate cancer risk.

Conclusion:
A Clinical Translational Approach

Inflammation involves a complex interaction of gene networks and is largely self-regulating, thus it is reasonable to assume that certain combinations of alleles may contribute to an imbalanced immune response and increased prostate cancer risk. Detection of prostate cancer in early stage is difficult, and current detection methods are inadequate. PSA testing is a significant advance for early diagnosis of patients with prostate cancer. PSA is mainly produced by prostate gland, and abnormalities of this organ are frequently associated with increased serum concentrations. Because of PSA's lack of specificity for prostate cancer, however, many patients undergo unnecessary biopsies or treatments for benign or latent tumours, respectively. Thus, other diagnostic approaches, such as identifying the pro-inflammatory profile of individuals will be helpful for diagnosis, prevention, and therapy. A major effort will be required to search a drug which interferes with the sequence of events triggered by the genetic mechanism(s) underlying this inflammatory age-related disease may be a good example of how genotyping is incorporated into clinical drug therapy in order to bridge the gap between pharmacogenetic research and clinical application. Macrophage-mediated antitumor effects could be augmented using TLR agonists, which have been shown to induce the regression of tumours through the engagement of both innate and adaptive immune systems [33].

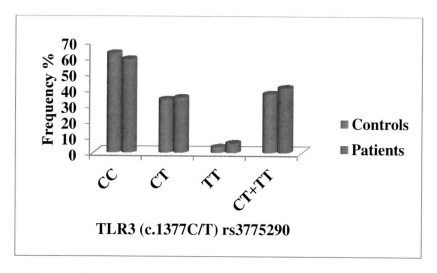

Figure 4. TLR3 gene variants and susceptibility to prostate cancer risk.

In addition, physicians and other health care providers need to be aware of this area of biomedical science in order to apply the information clinically. Different ethnicities may have different genetic backgrounds, which influence the prostate cancer susceptibility, so major effort should give to educate all members of the health care team about clinical genomics [34]. In long term perspective, the pharmacogenomic knowledge will help our pharmaceutical industry to develop drugs, which are more suited to the people of the country. Innate immune biology is a young field of medical research that holds much promise for risk stratification and novel therapeutic approaches. The innate immune receptors are involved in a large number of biological processes, and their study has uncovered individual susceptibility factors to numerous diseases. TLR expression appears to be an important factor in the biological pathogenesis of prostate cancer; however, as a series of candidate independent prognostic factors these markers may be confounded by variables such as Gleason score. Thus, anti-inflammatory agents should be explored for both prevention and treatment of cancer. Their true potential will be recognized only through well-controlled clinical trials.

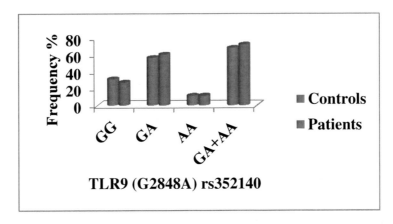

Figure 5. TLR9 gene variants and susceptibility to prostate cancer risk.

References

[1]   A. Jemal, R. Siegel, J. Xu, E. Ward, *CA Cancer J Clin. 5*, 277 (2010).

[2]   M. J. Hayat, N. Howlader, M. E. Reichman, B.K. Edwards, *Oncologist. 12*, 20 (2007).

[3]   P. Lichtenstein, N. V. Holm, P. K. Verkasalo, A. Iliadou, J. Kaprio, M. Koskenvuo, E. Pukkala, A. Skytthe, K. Hemminki, *N Engl J Med. 343*, 78 (2000).

[4]   C. Caruso, D. Lio, L. Cavallone, C. Franceschi, *Ann N Y Acad Sci. 1028*, 1 (2004).

[5]   P. Allavena, C. Garlanda, M. G. Borrello, A. Sica, A. Mantovani, *Curr Opin Genet Dev. 18*, 3 (2008).

[6]   D. G. Bostwick, G. Roza, P. Dundore, F. A. Corica, K. A. Iczkowski, *Prostate. 55*, 187 (2003).

[7]   G. Theyer, G. Kramer, I. Assmann, E. Sherwood, W. Preinfalk, M. Marberger, O. Zechner, G. E. Steine, *Lab Invest. 66*, 96 (1999).

[8]   R. J. Cohen, B. A. Shannon, J. E. McNeal, T. Shannon, K. L. Garrett, *J Urol. 173*, 1969 (2005).

[9]   R. Schlaberg, D. J. Choe, K. R. Brown, H. M. Thaker, I. R. Singh, *Proc Natl Acad Sci USA. 106*, 16351 (2009).

[10] R. B. Hayes, L. M. Pottern, H. Strickler, C. Rabkin, V. Pope, G. M. Swanson, R. S. Greenberg, J. B. Schoenberg, J. Liff, A. G. Schwartz, R. N. Hoover, J. F. Fraumeni, *Br J Cancer. 82*, 718 (2000).

[11] H. D. Strickler, J. J. Goedert, *Epidemiol Rev. 23*, 144 (2001).

[12] M. L. Taylor, A. G. Mainous, B. J. Wells, *Fam Med. 37*, 506 (2005).

[13] K. A. Rosenblatt, K. G. Wicklund, J. L. Stanford, *Am J Epidemiol. 153*, 1152 (2001).

[14] A. Zambrano, M. Kalantari, A. Simoneau, J. L. Jensen, L. P. Villarreal, *Prostate.* *53*, 263 (2002).

[15] M. Samanta, L. Harkins, K. Klemm, W. J. Britt, C. S. Cobbs, *J Urol.* *170*, 998 (2003).

[16] J. E. Mc. Neal, *Am J Surg Pathol.* *8*, 619 (1988).

[17] A. M. De. Marzo, V. L. Marchi, J. I. Epstein, W. G. Nelson, *Am J Pathol.* *155*, 1985 (1999).

[18] M. J. Putzi, A. M. De. Marzo, *Urology.* *56*, 828 (2000).

[19] D. Tomas, B. Kruslin, H. Rogatsch, G. Schäfer, M. Belicza, G. Mikuz, *Eur Urol.* *51*, 98 (2007).

[20] G. E. Steiner, B. Djavan, G. Kramer, Handisurya A, Newman M, C. Lee, M. Marberger, *Rev Urol.* *4*, 171 (2002).

[21] W. W. Hochreiter, R. B. Nadler, A. E. Koch, P. L. Campbell, M. Ludwig, Weidner W, A. J. Schaeffer. *Urology.* *56*, 1025 (2000).

[22] K. Fujita, C. M. Ewing, L. J. Sokoll, D. J. Elliott, M. Cunningham, A. M. De. Marzo, W. B. Isaacs, C. P. Pavlovich, *Prostate.* *68*, 872 (2008).

[23] K, Takeyama, H. Mitsuzawa, T, Shimizu, M. Konishi, C, Nishitani, H. Sano, Y, Kunishima, M, Matsukawa, S, Takahashi, K, Shibata, T, Tsukamoto, Y, Kuroki, *Prostate.* *66*, 386 (2006).

[24] B. R. Zysow, G. E. Lindahl, D. P. Wade, B. L. Knight, R. M. Lawn, *Arterioscler Thromb Vasc Biol.* *15*, 58 (1995).

[25] E. M. El-Omar, M. T. Ng, G. L. Hold, *Oncogene.* *27*, 244 (2008).

[26] R. K. Mandal, G. P. George, R. D. Mittal. *Mol Biol Rep.* *39*, 7263 (2012).

[27] S. D. Kundu, C. Lee, B. K. Billips, G. M. Habermacher, Q. Zhang, V. Liu, L. Y. Wong, D. J. Klumpp, P. Thumbikat, *Prostate.* *68*, 223 (2008).

[28] J. Sun, F. Wiklund, S. L. Zheng, B. Chang, K. Bälter, L. Li, J. E. Johansson, G. Li, H. O. Adami, W. Liu, A. Tolin, A. R. Turner, D. A. Meyers, W. B. Isaacs, J. Xu, H. Grönberg, *J Natl Cancer Inst.* *97*, 525 (2005).

[29] V. L. Stevens, A. W. Hsing, J. T. Talbot, S. L. Zheng, J. Sun, J. Chen, M. J. Thun, J. Xu, E. E. E. Calle, C. Rodriguez C, *Int J Cancer.* *123*, 2644 (2008).

[30] J. Xu, J. Lowey, F. Wiklund, J. Sun, F. Lindmark , F. C. Hsu, L. Dimitrov, B. Chang, A. r. Turner, W. Liu, H. O. Adami, E. Suh, J. H. Moore, S. L. Zheng, W. B. Isaacs, J. M. Trent, H. Grönberg, *Cancer Epidemiol Biomarkers Prev.* *14*, 2563 (2005).

[31] H. J. Kim, J. S. Bae, I. H. Chang, K. D. Kim, J. Lee, H. D. Shin, J.Y. Lee, W. J. Kim, W. Kim, S. C. Myung, *World J Urol.* *30*, 225 (2012).

[32] Y.C. Chen, E. Giovannucci, P. Kraft, R. Lazarus, D. J. Hunter, *Cancer Epidemiol Biomarkers Prev.* *16*, 1982 (2007).

[33] J. Vollmer, *Int Rev Immunol.* *25*, 125 (2006).

[34] L. Wang, H. L. Mc. Leod, R. M. Weinshilboum, *N Engl J Med.* *364*, 1144 (2011).

In: Handbook of Genitourinary Medicine: New Research   ISBN: 978-1-62618-226-4
Editor: Rashmi R. Singh   © 2013 Nova Science Publishers, Inc.

Chapter IV

Vesicoureteric Reflux

Andrew Moon, Nikhil Vasdev and *Andrew C. Thorpe*
Department of Urology, Freeman Hospital, Newcastle upon Tyne, UK

Abstract

Vesicoureteric reflux describes the retrograde flow of urine from the bladder into the collecting system of the kidneys. This condition predominantly affects young children and may be associated with urinary tract infections. In its most severe form a reflux nephropathy can develop causing hypertension and renal failure. Early diagnosis and close monitoring are integral to the management of VUR. Preventing urinary tract infection and permanent renal parenchymal damage underpins the treatment of those affected by VUR. Controversy still remains with regards to the optimal management strategies.

Introduction

Vesicoureteric reflux (VUR) describes the retrograde flow of urine from the bladder into the collecting system of the kidneys. This condition predominantly affects young children and may be associated with urinary tract infections (UTI). In its most severe form a reflux nephropathy can develop causing hypertension and renal failure.

Unrecognized VUR may lead to long-term effects on renal function and overall patient health. The severity of VUR varies greatly amongst patients. Early diagnosis and close monitoring are integral to the management of VUR.

Preventing urinary tract infection and permanent renal parenchymal damage underpins the treatment of those affected by VUR. Controversy still remains with regards to the optimal management strategies. [1,2]

---

* Correspondence – Mr Nikhil Vasdev, FRCS (Urol), Senior Specialist Registrar, Department of Urology, Freeman Hospital, Newcastle upon Tyne, UK.

Epidemiology

It is estimated that the prevalence of VUR in the general pediatric population is 1-2%. VUR occurs in 25 - 40% of children assessed following presentation with acute symptomatic UTI [3].

The incidence of prenatally diagnosed hydronephrosis caused by VUR varies from 17 – 34% [4,5]. Male newborns have a higher incidence of reflux, however as children get older, VUR affects girls five times more frequently than boys. VUR is ten times more common in Caucasian children and in those with red hair than in those of African American descent [6].

There also appears to be a strong genetic basis linked to the development of VUR. Twin and family studies suggest that the children of parents with VUR have a 70% risk of developing reflux. In addition, younger siblings of affected individuals have a 30% risk of being affected [7]. With the majority of VUR patients asymptomatic, relatives should be encouraged to attend for routine radiological screening for reflux. [8,9]

Embryology and Anatomy

The reflux of urine in healthy individuals is prevented by low bladder pressures and the occlusion of the distal ureter by the vesicoureteric junction (VUJ) during bladder contraction.

The normal valve mechanism of the VUJ is maintained by the oblique insertion of the intramural ureter, adequate length of the intramural segment of the ureter and strong detrusor muscle support. In addition, during bladder filling, the distal ureter is compressed against the muscular bladder wall. These features create a valvular mechanism at the VUJ preventing urinary reflux during bladder filling and voiding. The effectiveness of this anti-reflux mechanism is directly related to the intramural ureteric length [10,11].

Primary VUR is recognized as a congenital abnormality of the structure of the vesicoureteric junction. Such anatomical defects include shortening of the intravesical ureters, absence of detrusor muscle and the lateral displacement of the ureteral orifice. During bladder filling, there is failure of the valve like mechanism at the VUJ allowing the retrograde flow of urine [12].

The embryological development of the VUJ is important in developing an understanding of the principles of reflux disease. Ureteric and renal development are mediated by the formation of the ureteral bud from the mesonephric duct. This represents the final stage of renal development, forming the metanephric kidney. The mesonephric duct is absorbed into the developing bladder (urogenital sinus), during which the final location of the ureteral bud determines the position of the ureteral orifice. If the ureteral bud reaches the urogenital sinus too early, it is located more proximally and laterally in the bladder wall. This abnormal position of the ureteric bud is associated with VUR due to shortening of the intravesical ureteric length [13]. It is also associated with renal dysplasia. The origin of the ureteral bud is most likely genetically determined [11].

In normal, healthy patients, the intramural ureteric length to diameter ratio is 5:1. VUR occurs following congenital anatomical abnormalities resulting in shortening of the intramural ureter length – ratio < 5:1. Pacquin reports that refluxing ureters have an intramural tunnel length to ureteral diameter ratio of 1.4:1 [14]. Failure of this flap valve mechanism at the VUJ results in the abnormal backflow of urine.

In secondary causes of VUR, the valvular mechanism at the VUJ is initially intact and functioning, however elevated intravesical pressures associated with either anatomical or functional bladder outflow obstruction causes damage to the VUJ.

Anatomical: Posterior urethral valves; urethral or meatal stenosis. These causes are treated surgically when possible.

Functional: Bladder instability, neurogenic bladder and non-neurogenic neurogenic bladder UTIs may cause reflux due to the elevated intravesical pressures associated with inflammation. Resolution can occur if the underlying cause is treated - medical and/or surgical treatment may be indicated [12].

Classification of VUR

VUR is classified into 5 grades according to the International Reflux Grading system [15]. This system, first introduced in 1985, assesses the degree of retrograde filling and dilatation of the renal system based on the radiological appearances present on a voiding cystourethrogram (VCUG).

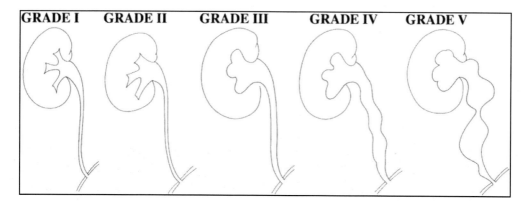

Figure 1. International Reflux Grading system.

- Grade I – retrograde filling of urine into ureter only
- Grade II – retrograde filling of urine into ureter, renal pelvis, and calyces
- Grade III – retrograde filling of urine into ureter and collecting system. Ureter and pelvis appear mildly dilated and the calyces are mildly blunted.
- Grade IV – retrograde filling of urine into ureter and collecting system. Ureter and pelvis appear moderately dilated and the calyces are moderately blunted.
- Grade V – retrograde filling of urine into ureter and collecting system. Severe dilatation of the pelvis, tortuous ureter appears tortuous and severe blunting of the calyces.

Presentation of VUR

VUR may be suspected but not diagnosed during prenatal ultrasound scanning when dilatation of the upper urinary tract is noted. It is estimated that 10% of these neonates will then be found to have vesicoureteric reflux postnatally [16].

Traditionally, VUR is asymptomatic, not causing any specific signs or symptoms unless complicated by febrile UTI. Clinical features in the paediatric patient may include irritability, pyrexia and lethargy or in the older child a history of urinary symptoms.

Undiagnosed VUR represents a significant cause of morbidity having long term implications. Patients with VUR are at an increased risk for pyelonephritis, hypertension and worsening renal failure.

Complications of VUR

It is estimated that 30-50% of children with symptomatic VUR have radiological evidence of renal scarring. These scars can be wedge shaped and are often associated with cortical thinning and distortion of the calyces. The renal damage may be the result of interstitial inflammation following the reflux of infected urine, mechanical damage following the high pressure reflux of sterile urine or abnormal embryological development causing renal dysplasia.

UTI is the most mportant risk factor for renal scarring. The retrograde flow of infected urine appears to stimulate the host's immune response causing fibrosis and renal scarring. This scarring is most commonly found at the renal poles during DMSA renal scanning.

The presence of renal scarring is often associated with higher grades of VUR and can result in serious hypertension following activation of the renin-angiotensin system. Reflux nephropathy is believed to be the most common cause of childhood hypertension. Studies suggest that $10 - 20\%$ of children affected by reflux nephropathy develop hypertension or end stage renal failure [17]. Wallace reports that hypertension develops in 10% of children with unilateral scars and 18.5% in those patients with bilateral scars. In addition, 4% of children with VUR progress to end stage renal failure [18].

The severity of VUR is varied and thus individuals are affected differently. In addition, some may have a genetic susceptibility to developing renal injury. VUR treatment modalities should consider resolution of reflux, cessation of UTIs and the function of the kidney.

Diagnosis

The early diagnosis and monitoring of VUR is key in the management of this disease process and from preventing its complications.

Initially, a detailed medical history including family history, physical examination, urinalysis and urine culture should be performed in all neonates born with pre or postnatal hydronephrosis to exclude UTI. Serum creatinine and electrolytes are also useful investigations to assess renal function.

Voiding cystourethrography (VCUG) or radionuclear cystourethrography (RNC) along with renal tract ultrasound scan should be performed in any child with a febrile UTI to confirm the diagnosis of VUR.

A dimercaptosuccinic acid (DMSA) renal scan can also be used to evaluate for renal abnormalities.

Until the resolution of VUR or the condition is treated surgically, the patient should undergo 12 – 24 month monitoring with cystography (RNC or VCUG). Annual ultrasonography may also be performed to monitor renal growth, detect hydronephrosis and to evaluate bladder anatomy and voiding dynamics.

There is also a role for urodynamics in those patients with secondary VUR caused by lower urinary tract dysfunction.

Cystoscopy was previously thought to be important during VUR assessment. The location of ureteral orifices was thought to correlate with VUR grade and prognosis. Subsequent studies have demonstrated that cystoscopic observations do not contribute significantly to the outcome of management [19].

Natural Progression of VUR

As a child grows, the intramural segment of the ureter lengthens, improving the competence of the VUJ valve mechanism. VUR, therefore, often resolves with increasing age. Primary VUR shows a tendency to improve in patients aged 6 - 10 years [20-24]. Normal renal growth can be expected in patients with VUR providing there are no further recurrent urinary tract infections.

The most important factor in the resolution of VUR is the severity of reflux. As the grade of VUR severity increases, the rate of spontaneous resolution diminishes [25,26] -

- Grade 1 : 85 – 92%
- Grade II : 63 – 76%
- Grade III : 53 – 62%
- Grade IV : 32 – 33%
- Grade V : < 10%

In addition, the duration of VUR in patients with higher grades is longer than in those with lower grades [21-24].

VUR Management Options

The ultimate aim of VUR management is to allow normal renal growth and to prevent permanent renal scarring and its associated complications. Resultantly, the early diagnosis of VUR and the subsequent monitoring of reflux and its complications is vital.

Treatment options for patients with VUR comprise conservative medical management and / or surgical intervention including open and laparoscopic correction of VUR or endoscopic injection.

The choice of therapy depends on the presence of renal scarring, the grade of reflux, renal function, bladder function and other abnormalities of the urinary tract, age, compliance with treatment and parental preference.

Medical Therapy

The rationale for conservative medical management is the observation that VUR can resolve spontaneously with time - mainly in young patients with low-grade reflux. Results from the International Reflux Study have identified that VUR patients can be managed conservatively with reduced risk of renal scarring provided urinary tract infections do not develop. There is increased likelihood of spontaneous resolution of VUR in children less than 5 years old with grades I-III reflux and in children younger than 1 year (especially boys). The higher grades of reflux (grades IV-V) may also resolve spontaneously providing they remain infection free [20-26].

The medical management of VUR is based upon the knowledge that low-grade reflux may resolve spontaneously and that the reflux of sterile urine does not damage the kidneys. Key aspects of conservative treatment include long term antibiotic prophylaxis, education, good fluid intake, bladder management including double voiding and lower urinary tract hygiene, managing the presence of voiding dysfunction and performing annual radiographic surveillance studies to assess the degree of reflux [11,19].

Continuous antibacterial prophylaxis decreases the incidence of pyelonephritis and subsequent renal scarring in patients with VUR. Voiding dysfunction including detrusor over activity can be a common cause of secondary VUR. There may also be a role for the use of anticholinergics in patients with poor bladder compliance and for circumcision in young male patients with low grade VUR [11,19].

Surgical Intervention

Relative indications for the surgical management of VUR include high grade and persistent reflux that is resistant to medical treatment, recurrent UTIs in patients on long term antibiotic prophylaxis, multiple drug allergies that prevent the use of antibiotics, a desire to stop antibiotic prophylaxis treatment and poor compliance with medical therapy [11,19].

Absolute indications for surgical management include the development of break through pyelonephritis, continued renal scarring despite antibiotic prophylaxis and an abnormal VUJ [11,19]. The surgical intervention of VUR may include open and laparoscopic surgical techniques or endoscopic injection. The definitive surgical treatment for primary VUR is ureteral reimplantation.

The principles required for successful reimplantation include :

- creating a long submucosal tunnel to provide a 5:1 tunnel-to-diameter ratio
- providing good detrusor muscle backing
- avoiding ureteric kinking

All VUR surgical techniques share this basic principle of lengthening the intramural part of the ureter by submucosal embedding of the ureter. This creates an effective flap-valve mechanism at the vesicoureteric junction. Current open surgical techniques have been shown to be safe with a low rate of complications and excellent success rates (92-98%) [2,27].

Laparoscopic reflux correction appears to be as successful as open techniques, however, does take significantly longer.

Endoscopic VUR treatment aims to inject a bulking agent below the intravesical portion of the ureter. This elevates the distal ureter and ureteral orifice, narrowing the lumen, thus preventing the backflow of urine. Endoscopic treatment offers the advantages of treating the anatomical defect whilst avoiding the risks associated with open surgery.

Recent data for endoscopic VUR management indicates that success rates at one year are significantly lower than initially reported, suggesting poor long-term outcomes for this technique [28].

Following surgical intervention, patients should undergo post-operative renal ultrasound scanning at 1 – 2 months and nuclear cystography at 3 months. Renal ultrasound scanning should then be performed annually for 3 years. Blood pressure measurement and urinalysis should be performed as a matter of routine during follow up. Once the resolution of VUR has been confirmed, antibiotic prophylaxis may be stopped.

A recent review of the International Reflux Study published the follow up results of patients 10 years after VUR intervention. The authors concluded that only a small number of patients developed new renal scarring and this occurred rarely after the first 5 years. They also identified that there was no difference between those treated medically or surgically [29].

At present, there are no long term studies comparing the efficacy of medical and surgical management or the surveillance monitoring of VUR. Outcome measures for all three modalities should consider not only resolution of VUR and the long-term implications on renal function and the recurrence of UTIs.

References

[1] Elder JS, Peters CA, Arant BS Jr, Ewalt DH, Hawtrey CE, Hurwitz RS, Parrott TS, Snyder HM 3rd,Weiss RA, Woolf SH, Hasselblad V. Pediatric Vesicoureteral Reflux Guidelines Panel summary report on the management of primary vesicoureteral reflux in children. *J Urol* 1997;157:1846-1851.

[2] Wheeler DM, Vimalachandra D, Hodson EM, Roy LP, Smith GH, Craig JC. Interventions for primary vesicoureteric reflux. *Cochrane Database Syst Rev* 2004;(3):CD001532.

[3] Fanos V, Cataldi L. Antibiotics or surgery for vesicoureteric reflux in children. *Lancet* 2004; 364 : 1720. 1722

[4] Anderson NG, Wright S, Abbott GD, Wells JE, Mogridge N. Fetal renal pelvic dilatation - poor predictor of familial vesicoureteric reflux. *Pediatr Nephrol* 2003;18:902-905.

[5] Phan V, Traubici J, Hershenfield B, Stephens D, Rosenblum ND, Geary DF. Vesicoureteral reflux in infants with isolated antenatal hydronephrosis. *Pediatr Nephrol* 2003;18:1224-1228.

[6] Mattoo TK. Vesicoureteral reflux and reflux nephropathy. *Adv Chronic Kidney Dis.* 2011 Sep;18(5):348-54.

[7] Murawski IJ, Gupta IR. Vesicoureteric reflux and renal malformations: a developmental problem. *Clin Genet* 2006;69:105-117.

[8] Hollowell JG, Greenfield SP. Screening siblings for vesicoureteral reflux. *J Urol* 2002;168:2138-2141.

[9] Giel DW, Noe HN, Williams MA. Ultrasound screening of asymptomatic siblings of children with vesicoureteral reflux: a long-term followup study. *J Urol* 2005;174:1602-1604.

[10] Bollgren I, Winberg J. The periurethral flora in girls highly susceptible to urinary infections. *Acta Pediatr Scand* 1976; 65: 81-87.

[11] Belman AB. Vesicoureteric reflux. *Pediatr Clin N Am* 1997; 44: 1171-1190.

[12] Reynard J, Brewster S, Biers S, *Oxford Handbook of Urology* Second Edition, pages 626 – 627.

[13] Avner E, Harmon W, Niaudet P, Yoshikawa N. *Paediatric Nephrology* Sixth Edition, Chapter 55 – Vesiocureteral reflux and renal scarring.

[14] Paquin AJ, Zinner NR, Arbuckle LD. Mechanical factors influencing the demonstrability of vesiocureteric reflux. *Am J Surg* 107, 492-496.

[15] Lebowitz RL, Olbing H, Parkkulainen KV, Smellie JM, Tamminen-Mobius TE. International Reflux Study in Children: international system of radiographic grading of vesicoureteric reflux. *Pediatr Radiol* 1985;15:105-109.

[16] Rosenberg AR, Kainer G, Srivastava T, Hughes C, Leighton O, Garrett W, *et al..* Long term followup of minimal collecting system dilatation detected in antenatal period. *Pediatr Nephrol1995*; 9: C 26.

[17] Blumenthal I. Vesicoureteric reflux and urinary tract infection in children. Postgrad Med J 2006;82:31-35.

[18] Wallace DMA, Rothwell DL, Williams DI et al.:The long term follow up of surgically treated vesicoureteric reflux. *Br J Urol* 50: 479, 1978.

[19] Elder JS. Guidelines for consideration for surgical repair of vesicoureteric reflux. *Curr Opin Urol* 2000;10:579-585.

[20] Linshaw M. Asymptomatic bacteriuria and vesicoureteral reflux in children. *Kidney Int* 1996; 50: 312-329.

[21] Arant BS Jr. Medical management of mild and moderate vesicoureteral reflux: Followup studies of infants and young children. A preliminary report of the Southwest Pediatric Nephrology Group. *J Urol* 1992; 148: 1683-1687.

[22] Huang F-Y, Tsai T-C. Resolution of vesicoureteral reflux during medical management of children. *Pediatr Nephrol* 1995; 9: 715-717.

[23] Vernon SJ, Coulthard MG, Lambert HJ, Keir MJ, Mathews JN. New renal scarring in children who at age 3 and 4 years had normal scans with dimercaptosuccinic acid: Follow up study. *Br Med J* 1997; 315: 905-908.

[24] Goldraich NP, Goldraich IH. Followup of conservatively treated children with high and low grade vesicoureteral reflux study. *J Urol* 1992; 148: 1688-1692.

[25] Arant BS Jr. Medical management of mild and moderate vesicoureteral reflux: followup studies of infants and young children. A preliminary report of the Southwest Pediatric Nephrology Study Group. *J Urol* 1992;148:1683-1687.

[26] Smellie JM, Jodal U, Lax H, Mobius TT, Hirche H, Olbing H; Writing Committee, International Reflux Study in Children (European Branch). Outcome at 10 years of severe vesicoureteric reflux managed medically: report of the International Reflux Study in Children. *J Pediatr* 2001;139:656-663.

[27] Birmingham Reflux Study Group: Prospective trial of operative versus non operative treatment of severe vesicoureteric reflux in children: Five years observation. *Br Med J Clin Res Edu* 1987; 295: 237- 241.

[28] Ritchey ML, Bloom D. Report of the American Academy of Pediatrics Section of Urology Meeting. *Pediatr Nephrol* 1995; 9: 642-646.

[29] Olbing H, Smellie JM, Jodal U, Lax H. New renal scars in children with severe VUR: a 10-year study of randomized treatment. *Pediatr Nephrol* 2003;18:1128-1131.

In: Handbook of Genitourinary Medicine: New Research
Editor: Rashmi R. Singh
ISBN: 978-1-62618-226-4
© 2013 Nova Science Publishers, Inc.

Chapter V

Genetic Models for Genitourinary Malformations

Irina B. Grishina[*]
Department of Urology, New York University School of Medicine,
New York, NY, US

Abstract

Defects in development of embryonic cloaca range from cloacal and bladder exstrophy, imperforate anus and rectourethral or rectovaginal fistula, to scrotal, penile and glandular hypospadias in the male. The current text-book concepts of cloacal development are based largely on anatomical studies conducted since 1850s. However valuable, these anatomic and histological observations are necessarily descriptive and, thus, limited in their capacity to identify the etiology of urologic defects. This chapter provides an overview how this problem is resolved by employing genetic rodent models. Genetically modified mice provide excellent tools for analysis of gene and cell lineage functions in urologic development and malformations. This review will outline the progress and perspectives of genetic mouse models in analysis of urologic malformations.

1. Embryology of Cloacal Development

The embryonic cloacal cavity is defined when the endodermal epithelium of the hindgut comes in contact with the ectoderm anterior to the tail [1-5]. This important caudal patterning event takes place at about 3 weeks of gestation age (GA)[2] in human and at embryonic day 9.5 (E9.5) in the mouse. At subsequent embryonic stages cloacal epithelium and mesenchyme undergo complex morphogenesis to give rise to the urinary bladder, urethra, genital tubercle and the rectum [6-9]. During sexually naïve stages, in between E10.5 to E14.0 in the mouse and during 4 to 8 weeks GA in human, the dorsal/rectal and ventral/urinary compartments

---

[*] Irina.grishina@nyumc.org, grishina.irina@gmail.com.

become topologically separate with own external orifices. The initial genital tubercle formation also takes place in this period. Cloacal and genital region patterning at these stages is regulated by the caudal homeobox genes of the Hox9 – Hox13 paralogous groups [10-11], and by cell communications between the epithelium and mesenchyme mediated by signaling by the Sonic hedgehog (Shh), Bone morphogenetic proteins (Bmp), Fibroblast growth Factors (Fgf) and Wnts [1, 6, 8, 12-25]. Starting at E14.5 in mice and about 9 week GA in human, the urethra and external genitalia undergo sex specific differentiation driven by androgen signaling in the male [26-30].

2. Mechanistic Theories of Urologic Development

The early vertebrate phyla including fishes, reptiles, birds and the early mammals, Monotremes, retain a common cloacal opening for the urinary tract and digestive system during adult stages [31]. In contrast, in the later, Therian mammals, including Marsupials [3] and Placental, embryonic cloaca is separated in embryogenesis into the rectal and urinary systems [32, 33]. Cloacal and genital birth defects are very common in all mammals. Urogenital malformations are the second most common type of congenital defects in human. Severe urological malformations often present multi-systemic defects in the structure of the urethra, rectum, bladder, genitalia and the body wall. Such pediatric patients present with rectourethral and rectovaginal fistulas, bladder and cloacal extrophy, epispadias, and scrotal and perineal hyposapdias [19, 34-39]. These conditions often require multiple rounds of surgical corrections with variable outcomes. Even mild urologic defects, such as hypospadias in the male (an abnormal ventral position of the urethral opening in the phallus) can severely affect persons reproductive health and quality of life.

Original concepts and theories for cloacal development were derived from anatomical observations in children and human fetuses documented since 1830s [40 and references therein]. These studies were followed by analysis of spontaneous urologic malformations in domestic animals [41-42]. Anatomic and histologic studies built a very important foundation for our understanding of urologic tissue development. However these studies are necessarily descriptive and significantly challenged in defining cellular and molecular causes for malformations. A significant step forward was achieved with development of laboratory rodent models that allow precise embryo staging and stage-specific cellular and molecular analysis of urologic tissues. Rodent models were also instrumental in defining the effects of environmental agents on urologic development, including the modulators of Retinoic Acid and sex-specific steroid hormones pathways. The next advancement came with implementation of heterologous epithelial/mesenchymal graft analysis by T McNeal and G Cunha who discovered and emphasized the importance of mesenchymal paracrine signals for urothelial cell fate choice [43 and references therein]. These concepts have been amplified with development of genetically modified mice that allowed to explore cellular functions of these paracrine signals. Advances in genetic mouse engineering in the past decade enabled development of several useful conditional and genetic labeling systems to manipulate gene functions in a time and tissue-specific manner, and to trace the fate and migration of specific cell lineages. Following is a summary of the current theories for cloacal development and the recent experimental data in their support.

1. *The rostro-caudal mesenchymal growth hypothesis.* The early anatomical studies in human and animal models [41, 42, 44-45] postulated that the driving factor for cloacal partioning is caudal growth of the axial cloacal mesenchyme defined as the "urorectal septum". Altough some of the studies questioned the existence of urorectal septum as a morphologic unit [46 and references therein], genetic studies in Shh models provide a measure of support for this theory. Authors showed that Shh expressed in cloacal endoderm induces high rate of cell proliferation in adjacent periurthral mesenchyme in effect promoting growth of the septum [21, 23].

2. *The axial constriction hypothesis.* Hynes and Fraher [2-4] performed a thorough histological analysis of cloacal partitioning and early genital extension in the mouse. Authors proposed that septation is driven by axial constriction of lateral mesenchyme. It would be very interesting to test this model using mesenchymal cell lineage tracing..

3. *Regulation of progenitor cell survival hypothesis.* A spontaneous mutation in the Danforth's short-tail mouse produces a rectourethral fistula in homozygotes that is accompanied by a loss of dorsal cloacal tissues [44-45]. Sasaki et al.. [5] showed a role for limited programmed cell death in the process of cloacal partitioning. We showed that exsessive cell death can deplete cloacal progenitor cell pool and contribute to a failure to form a septal plate [25].

4. *Endodermal remodeling hypothesis.* Our genetic studies in mouse models indicate that cloacal partitioning requires Bmp signaling that promotes formation of the septal plate by inducing apical-basal orientation of cell divisions in the cloacal epithelium.

Notably, altough these hypothesis focus on different tissue remodeling aspects of cloacal septaion, the majority of experimental data point to the role of signaling mechanisms in regulating various aspects of the cell division cycle.

3. Caudal Homeobox Models

Genetic studies indicate that caudal homeobox genes, from Hox9 to Hox13 paralogous groups, function to pattern the cloacal region, and that mutations in these genes cause caudal deffects similar across mammalian species. The *Hoxa13* and *Hoxd13* are expressed in the cloacal area and are essential for morphogenesis of all cloacal derivatives both in human, and in murine models [10, 47-50]. Dominant negative mutation of the *Hoxa13* is the cause of the Hand-Foot-Genital Syndrome in human [48-50]. In the mouse, limb and genital malformations similar to Hand-Foot-Genital Syndrome have been described in the mouse hypolydactyly model, *Hoxa13$^{Hd/Hd}$*, resulting from a 50 bp deletion in the *Hoxa13* gene. A similar Synpolydactyly Syndrome in human results from a dominant negative mutation in *Hoxd13* and manifests in digit fusions and hypospadias [51]. This *Hoxd13* mutation also results in digit and genital phenotype in the mouse [52]. In turn, *Hoxa13$^{-/-}$;Hoxd13$^{-/-}$* mouse mutants show severe genital and cloacal malformations [10]. *Hoxa13-/-* null embryos develop hypospadia and show a ventrally positioned anus [11]. *Hoxd13* and *Hoxd12* mutations in the mouse result in disorganized anal sphincter muscle [52]. The *Hlxb9,* is the major candidate for another caudal syndrom, the Curarino [53]. The Hox genes transcriptional targtes in caudal development are not yet clear. However, studies point to several signaling factors, in particular, Bmps, Bmp repressor Noggin, and Fgf8 [11]. In turn, studies in rodent models indicate that several environmental agents can cause caudal defects by interfering with the retinoic acid pathway that regulates caudal Hox gene time and expression domains. Administration of retinoic acid at late gastrulation results in an anterior shift in the *Hox10 – Hox13* expression domains [54-55] and results in cloacal defects. Later administration of retinoic acid leads to hypospadias [56]. Hox are not the only homeobox genes contributing to caudal patterning. Others include the Dlx and Tbx factors [19, 57].

4. Bmp and Noggin Models

4.1. Early Establishment of Cloacal Tissues

Shortly after gastrulation, the primitive gut forms an attachment to the ectoderm at site of the late primitive streak, called the ventral ectodermal ridge (VER). The Bmp/Noggin axis plays a crucial role in regulating cell and tissue content during cloacal region formation. Prior to cloacal formation Bmps are expressed in the VER. Signaling by Bmp2, Bmp4 and Bmp7 expressed in the VER functions to promote epithelial to mesenchymal transition (EMT) to supply the pericloacal mesoderm. Timely cessation of EMT is regulated by the Bmp inhibitor Noggin [58-59]. *Noggin* null mutants fail to properly develop caudal cloacal derivatives, the rectum, perineal urethra and genital appendage. In addition, Bmp7 functions in partitioning of the cloaca into the urethral and rectal compartments [8, 25]. Together, these studies underline the importance of the Bmp pathway at multiple stages in urologic development, and indicate that deregulation of signaling at various developmental stages can cause a range of cloacal and genital malformations.

Cloacal malformations are a part of a larger group of caudal deformities defined as the caudal regression syndrome (CRS). Important common feature of the CRS is the multiple defects in the ventral midline that includes bladder, genitalia and body wall. Mutant embryos manifest cloacal and bladder exstrophies, and often display fusion of both hindlimbs called sirenomelia, or the mermaid phenotype [58-59]. CRS has been traced to deregulation of the Bmp/Noggin axis at the late gastrula stage [57-61]. Under Bmp signal, cells from the VER undergo EMT and supply pericloacal mesenchyme [57-58]. Combined loss of *Bmp7* and *Twisted gastrulation* genes [60], or *Bmp7* alone in *C3H* mouse strain background (our unpublished data), results in severe defects in the ventral midline, in particular, loss of the bladder and sirenomelia. Induction of the EMT in the VER is mediated by the Smad1/5/8 factors that activate expression of the Snail/Slug genes that downregulate transcription of E-cadherin [58]. In addition, Bmps function in the VER to promote expression of metalloproteinases that degrade the basal membrane [62]. The end of gastrulation that stops supply of the caudal mesoderm is regulated by increase in *Noggin* [58-59]. Increase in Noggin in caudal mesenchyme leads to stabilization of the ectoderm basal membrane and cessation of the EMT.

Genital ectoderm continues to express Bmp ligands through the course of cloacal and genital development [8, 11, 18]. Genetic inactivation of *Noggin* results in continuation of the EMT until depletion of VER. Consistently, *Noggin-/-* embryos show increased pericloacal mesenchyme and defects in epithelial structure of both the caudal hindgut and ectoderm [59]. In contrast, genetic inactivation of the *Bmp4* ligand results in insufficient mesoderm and lethality at gastrulation [63].

The VER contributes to the ectodermal part of the cloacal membrane and the ectoderm overlaying the genital appendage [8, 58]. Lineage tracing studies showed that pericloacal mesenchyme contributes to the genital appendage, bladder and the body wall [6, 58]. The *Noggin* null embryos show an increase in the tail mesenchyme, and a visible cytological disorganization of the ventral ectoderm and the gut endoderm [58]. Importantly, *Noggin-/-* embryos fail to form the attachment of the caudal hindgut to the ectoderm [58]. Formation of the gut-ectoderm contact and the cloacal membrane requires function of another signaling molecule, *Wnt5a,* which is expressed in the ventral ectodermal ridge and adjacent mesenchyme [21].

Wnt5a mutants show variable cloacal defects. In the most severe cases, the gut fails to make a contact with the ventral ectodermal ridge, and a blind cloacal pouch is found rostrally to its normal position. *Wnt5a* is one of the non-canonical Wnt molecules which signal through the Ror receptor and activate the c-Jun N-terminal kinase and Rho kinases [64-65]. *Noggin-/-* [58, 66], *Wnt5a-/-* [21, 67] and *Bmp7-/-;C3H* (our unpublished data) mutants show very similar defects in cloacal development and lack external genitalia. Bmps, in particular, Bmp4, can repress expression of *Wnt5a* in the genital mesenchyme [18]. Thus, it is likely that *Wnt5a* expression is positively regulated by the Noggin during cloacal development. Analysis of the *Noggin-/-* embryos shows lack of the perineal urethra, rectum and external genitalia [66]. Instead, the urogenital sinus and hindgut drain into a blind cloacal pouch. Interestingly, *Noggin-/-* mutants develop a functional bladder and most of prostate lobes [66]. Thus, Noggin function is specifically required for caudal organ development adjacent to the cloacal membrane.

4.2. Cloacal Partitioning

During normal fetal development, cloacal cavity separates axially into a ventral/urethral and dorsal/rectal compartments (Fig. 1A). Signaling communications between the mesenchyme and epithelium, in particular, those delivered by Bmps are for cloacal septation and early genital development [8, 25]. *Bmp7* null embryos show arrest in cloacal septation and form a rectourethral fistula by birth. We have shown that most of Bmp7 signaling in the cloacal region is mediated by the c-Jun N-terminal kinase (JNK) pathway [25]. Bmp/JNK signaling promotes increased cell proliferation in cloacal endodermal epithelium and mesenchyme, and signal is required for cell survival in the endoderm. Loss of *Bmp7* results in a dramatic increase in cell death in the dorsal and axial cloacal endoderm that normally forms the rectum and perineum [25].

Loss of *Bmp7* function results in atrophic rectum [8]. JNK kinases regulate various aspects of the cell division cycle, including cell proliferation, programmed cell death and polarity of cell divisions. The later is dependent on the JNK ability to stabilize the microtubule scaffold [68-69].

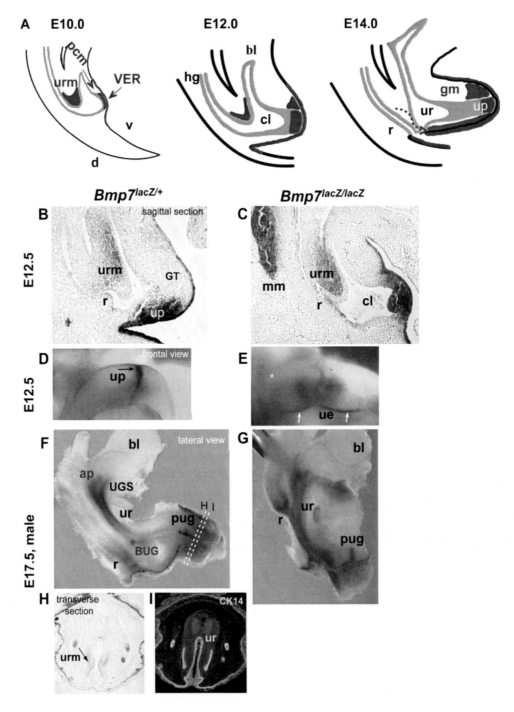

Figure 1. Bmp7 is important for cloacal septation and for morphogenesis of the genital urethra. (A) Time-line of cloacal partitioning in the mouse: endoderm (green), *Bmp7*^{lacZ} expression (blue). Bladder, bl; cloaca, cl; dorsal, d; hg, hindgut; genital, gm, pericloacal, pcm, and urorectal, urm, mesenchymal compartments; r, rectum; urethral plate; up; ventral, v; ventral ectodermal ridge, VER. At E12-14, *Bmp7* expression shifts from the urm to the ventral part of the genital tubercle (dashed arrow). (B-I) *Bmp7*^{lacZ} tissues are stained with X-gal (5-bromo-4-chloro-indolyl-β-D-galactopyranoside, blue). (B) Axial sagittal section of E12.5 *Bmp7*$^{lacZ/+}$ cloacal region shows normal partitioning into the rectal and

urethral compartments. (C) E12.5 *Bmp7* null cloacal cavity is extended and fails to septate. *Bmp7*-positive urm extends from the metanephric mesenchyme (mm). (D, E) Frontal views of a normal *Bmp7*$^{lacZ/+}$ (D) and *Bmp7* null (E) genital tubercle at E12.5. *Bmp7* null urethral plate unzipps ventrally (ue, urethral epithelium, arrows). (F) Lateral view of a normal male lower urogenital system at E17.5. *Bmp7* is expressed in epithelial and mesenchymal tissues, including the emerging buds of the bulbourethral gland (BUG), anterior prostate (AP), and preputial gland (pug). Dashed lines indicate the planes of transverse sections in H and I. (G) *Bmp7* null male embryo at E17.5 shows a rectourethral fistula and lacks BUG. (H, I) More proximal (H) and adjacent distally (I) sections of *Bmp7*$^{lacZ/+}$ male genital tubercle. (H) *Bmp7* (blue) is expressed in the mesenchyme flanking the fusion of the ventral urethra. (I) Urethral duct is visualized by labeling for cytokeratin 14 (CK14).

As we will show further, disruption of cell polarity in cloacal epithelium has important reprecautions for cloacal septation [25]. First, *Bmp7* null cloacal epithelium retains a simple cuboidal structure akin to primitive gut endoderm. The normal cloacal epithelium at these stages would have already formed stacked (stratified) epithelial layers [2-4, 8, 25]. Stratification requires an enforcement of epithelial cytoskeleton rigidity with specific intermediate filaments such as cytokeratin 14. Deficiency for *Bmp7* results in a lack of cytokeratin 14 expression at cloacal septation stages and as a result a simple cuboidal epithelial structure [25]. In addition, *Bmp7* null epithelium shows a significant abnormality in polarity of cell divisions. During normal cloacal septation the majority of cell divisions are polarized in the apical-basal direction [25]. In contrast, in the *Bmp7* null epithelium, cell divisions are randomized. During normal cloacal development, cloacal duct develops multilayered epithelial walls and a progressive narrowing of the lumen at axial position resulting in a septal plate [25]. Formation of this septal plate is directed by a mechanism favoring apical-basal orientation of cell divisions downstream of the Bmp7/JNK pathway. Namely, Bmp7 signaling from the urorectal mesenchyme activates JNK in the endoderm and promotes apical-basal polarity of cell divisions so that daughter cells extend along the length of the septal lumen allowing topological separation of the rectum and urethra.

Notably, the urorectal mesenchyme is also a target for Bmp7 signals that lead to activation of JNK and increase in cell proliferation. Deficiency for mesenchymal JNK activity can account for the loss of ventral genital structures in Bmp7 deficient embryos (Figure 1G). Further studies are important to define Bmp/JNK function in genital development. For example, this signaling pathway can regulate mesenchymal cell migration and contribute to formation of the corpus cavernosum urethrae [8]. Bmp signaling pathway is likely an evolutionary conserved mechanism of cloacal partitioning. For instance, Bmp signaling is required for cloacal partitioning in the zebrafish [70] where Bmp signal is mediated by the *HrT* gene, an ortholog of murine *T-box factor 20* [57].

4.3. Differentiation of the Genital Urethra

Initial stages of genital development, from E11 to E15 in the mouse, are gender-independent. Development of the genital appendage, the precursor of penis in males and clitoris in females, begins with appearance of genital swellings laterally to the cloaca at E10.5 [1, 20]. Bmp7 is important for initiation of genital urethra development. Null embryos show early defects in the uretral plate adhesion that results in unfolding of the plate (Figure 1E compare to D) and development of scrotal hypospadias (Figure 1G). Studies in human also show correlation between hypospadias and genetic variations in Bmp4 and Bmp7 alleles [71, 72].

Sexual differentiation of the genital urethra in the male is under the control of androgens secreted by the testis starting at about E15.5 in the mice [28, 29]. During normal male development, the urethral plate is canalized to form the urethral duct (Figure 1H, I). Then, ventral part of the urethra is fused starting from proximal to distal regions of the appendage (Figure 1H, I). In this process, ventral urethral seam is displaced by mesenchyme (Figure 1H; 2-4, 20].

Lineage labeling showed that urethral epithelial seam cells do not contribute to genital mesenchyme [20]. Thus, urethral remodeling does not involve epithelial to mesenchymal transition. In turn, mesenchymal lineage tracing showed that mesenchyme displacing ventral urethral seam originates from the Bmp7-expressing urorectal region and, presumably, migrates first caudally to the perineum and then distally along the ventral side of the genital tubercle [8].

5. Wnt Models

Canonical and non canonical Wnt signals are also important at multiple stages of cloacal and genital development. First, caudal position of the cloaca and its attachment to the ventral ectodermal ridge depends on non canonical Wnt5 [21].

Precise regulation of the canonical Wnt/beta-catenin pathway is also essential for early genital development [14]. During urethral remodeling, several important signaling mediators including androgen receptor, *Bmp4* and *Bmp7,* and several Wnt molecules are expressed in the mesenchyme flanking genital urethra [8, 11, 14, 16, 73]. Recent studies show that Wnt signaling is directly involved in genital masculinization by collaborating with the androgen receptor pathway [17]. During genital differentiation in females, or in androgen signaling deficient males, genital mesenchyme produces higher levels of Wnt inhibitors, Dkk2 and Sfrp1. As a result, in the developing male genitalia, canonical Wnt signaling is considerably higher then in females. The cellular effects of Wnt signals in remodeling of the genital urethra and/or the adjacent mesenchyme are still unknown.

Finally, Tbx20, the candidate coordinator for cloacal septation, regulates expression of several non-canonical Wnt mediators including a trans-membrane receptor component, *van Gogh 2 (Vangl2)* [74-75]. Examinations of mouse embryos hypomorphic for *Vangl2*, revealed multiple rectourethral and genital abnormalities including anal stenosis, genital hypospadias, and a decrease in anogenital distance (our unpublished data). Thus, future studies are important to define the coordinated canonical and non canonical Wnt functions at various stages of cloacal and genital development.

4. Shh and Fgf Models

Deficiencies in signaling by the Sonic Hedgehog (Shh) pathway, affect development of all components of the lower urethral system, including the bladder and external genitalia [6, 13, 46]. The graded reduction in Shh signaling in the *Shh* and *Gli2,3* mouse mutants recapitulates the whole range of cloacal and genital malformations in human [6, 13, 15, 21, 46]. In support of the Shh role in human disease, a portion of patients with Pallister-Hall syndrome, caused by a frameshift mutation in the Shh mediator, *Gli3*, present with rectourethral fistulas [69].

Shh is expressed in the caudal endoderm and functions in urologic organ development either by establishing mesenchymal patterning and/or by regulating patterned progenitor maintenance [6, 13, 76]. Lineage studies indicate that all urethral epithelim develops from the cloacal endoderm patterned by *Shh* [20]. Shh signaling in mid-embryogenesis plays a role in cloacal septaion [22]. In turn, during sexual differentiation, interactions between Shh, Wnt and androgen signaling s promote are important for urethral growth and formation of the tubular genital urethra in the male [15-16, 22].

In summary, studies in genetic mouse models have a significant potential to uncover cellular and molecular mechanisms of cloacal region development in the nearest future, and to add significantly to our understanding of the etiology of cloacal malformations.

References

[1]   Perriton CL, Powles N, Chiang C, Maconochie MK, Cohn MJ. Sonic hedgehog signaling from the urethral epithelium controls external genital development. *Dev Biol.* 2002 Jul 1;247(1):26-46.

[2]   Hynes PJ, Fraher JP. The development of the male genitourinary system: II. The origin and formation of the urethral plate. *Br J Plast Surg.* 2004 Mar;57(2):112-21.

[3]   Hynes PJ, Fraher JP. The development of the male genitourinary system: III. The formation of the spongiose and glandar urethra. *Br J Plast Surg.* 2004 Apr;57(3):203-14.

[4]   Hynes PJ, Fraher JP. The development of the male genitourinary system. I. The origin of the urorectal septum and the formation of the perineum. *Br J Plast Surg.* 2004 Jan;57(1):27-36.

[5]   Haraguchi R, Motoyama J, Sasaki H, Satoh Y, Miyagawa S, Nakagata N, et al.. Molecular analysis of coordinated bladder and urogenital organ formation by Hedgehog signaling. *Development.* 2007 Feb;134(3):525-33.

[6]   Ogi H, Suzuki K, Ogino Y, Kamimura M, Miyado M, Ying X, et al.. Ventral abdominal wall dysmorphogenesis of Msx1/Msx2 double-mutant mice. *Anat Rec A Discov Mol Cell Evol Biol.* 2005 May;284(1):424-30.

[7]   Wu X, Ferrara C, Shapiro E, Grishina I. Bmp7 expression and null phenotype in the urogenital system suggest a role in re-organization of the urethral epithelium. *Gene Expr Patterns.* 2009 Apr;9(4):224-30.

[8]   Shapiro E. Update on fetal surgery: highlights from the society for pediatric urology 49th annual meeting april 29, 2000, atlanta. *Rev Urol.* 2000 Fall;2(4):206-10.

[9]   Sasaki C, Yamaguchi K, Akita K. Spatiotemporal distribution of apoptosis during normal cloacal development in mice. Anat Rec A Discov *Mol Cell Evol Biol.* 2004 Aug;279(2):761-7.

[10] Warot X, Fromental-Ramain C, Fraulob V, Chambon P, Dolle P. Gene dosage-dependent effects of the Hoxa-13 and Hoxd-13 mutations on morphogenesis of the

terminal parts of the digestive and urogenital tracts. *Development.* 1997 Dec;124(23):4781-91.

[11] Morgan EA, Nguyen SB, Scott V, Stadler HS. Loss of Bmp7 and Fgf8 signaling in Hoxa13-mutant mice causes hypospadia. *Development.* 2003 Jul;130(14):3095-109.

[12] Haraguchi R, Suzuki K, Murakami R, Sakai M, Kamikawa M, Kengaku M, et al.. Molecular analysis of external genitalia formation: the role of fibroblast growth factor (Fgf) genes during genital tubercle formation. *Development.* 2000 Jun;127(11):2471-9.

[13] Haraguchi R, Mo R, Hui C, Motoyama J, Makino S, Shiroishi T, et al.. Unique functions of Sonic hedgehog signaling during external genitalia development. *Development.* 2001 Nov;128(21):4241-50.

[14] Lin C, Yin Y, Long F, Ma L. Tissue-specific requirements of beta-catenin in external genitalia development. *Development.* 2008 Aug;135(16):2815-25.

[15] Miyagawa S, Moon A, Haraguchi R, Inoue C, Harada M, Nakahara C, et al.. Dosage-dependent hedgehog signals integrated with Wnt/beta-catenin signaling regulate external genitalia formation as an appendicular program. *Development.* 2009 Dec;136(23):3969-78.

[16] Lin C, Yin Y, Veith GM, Fisher AV, Long F, Ma L. Temporal and spatial dissection of Shh signaling in genital tubercle development. *Development.* 2009 Dec;136(23):3959-67.

[17] Miyagawa S, Satoh Y, Haraguchi R, Suzuki K, Iguchi T, Taketo MM, et al.. Genetic interactions of the androgen and Wnt/beta-catenin pathways for the masculinization of external genitalia. *Mol Endocrinol.* 2009 Jun;23(6):871-80.

[18] Suzuki K, Bachiller D, Chen YP, Kamikawa M, Ogi H, Haraguchi R, et al.. Regulation of outgrowth and apoptosis for the terminal appendage: external genitalia development by concerted actions of BMP signaling [corrected]. *Development.* 2003 Dec;130(25):6209-20.

[19] Suzuki K, Haraguchi R, Ogata T, Barbieri O, Alegria O, Vieux-Rochas M, et al.. Abnormal urethra formation in mouse models of split-hand/split-foot malformation type 1 and type 4. *Eur J Hum Genet.* 2008 Jan;16(1):36-44.

[20] Seifert AW, Harfe BD, Cohn MJ. Cell lineage analysis demonstrates an endodermal origin of the distal urethra and perineum. *Dev Biol.* 2008 Jun 1;318(1):143-52.

[21] Seifert AW, Bouldin CM, Choi KS, Harfe BD, Cohn MJ. Multiphasic and tissue-specific roles of sonic hedgehog in cloacal septation and external genitalia development. *Development.* 2009 Dec;136(23):3949-57.

[22] Seifert AW, Yamaguchi T, Cohn MJ. Functional and phylogenetic analysis shows that Fgf8 is a marker of genital induction in mammals but is not required for external genital development. *Development.* 2009 Aug;136(15):2643-51.

[23] Seifert AW, Zheng Z, Ormerod BK, Cohn MJ. Sonic hedgehog controls growth of external genitalia by regulating cell cycle kinetics. *Nat Commun.* 2010;1:23.

[24] Petiot A, Perriton CL, Dickson C, Cohn MJ. Development of the mammalian urethra is controlled by Fgfr2-IIIb. *Development.* 2005 May;132(10):2441-50.

[25] Xu K, Wu X, Shapiro E, Huang H, Zhang L, Hickling D, et al.. Bmp7 functions via a polarity mechanism to promote cloacal septation. *PLoS One.* 2012;7(1):e29372.

[26] Drews U, Sulak O, Schenck PA. Androgens and the development of the vagina. *Biol Reprod.* 2002 Oct;67(4):1353-9.

[27] Kim KS, Liu W, Cunha GR, Russell DW, Huang H, Shapiro E, et al.. Expression of the androgen receptor and 5 alpha-reductase type 2 in the developing human fetal penis and urethra. *Cell Tissue Res.* 2002 Feb;307(2):145-53.

[28] Yucel S, Cavalcanti AG, Wang Z, Baskin LS. The impact of prenatal androgens on vaginal and urogenital sinus development in the female mouse. *J Urol.* 2003 Oct;170(4 Pt 1):1432-6.

[29] Yucel S, Liu W, Cordero D, Donjacour A, Cunha G, Baskin LS. Anatomical studies of the fibroblast growth factor-10 mutant, Sonic Hedge Hog mutant and androgen receptor mutant mouse genital tubercle. *Adv Exp Med Biol.* 2004;545:123-48.

[30] Buckley J, Willingham E, Agras K, Baskin LS. Embryonic exposure to the fungicide vinclozolin causes virilization of females and alteration of progesterone receptor expression in vivo: an experimental study in mice. *Environ Health.* 2006;5:4.

[31] Griffith M. 1978 *The Biology of the Monotremes.*

[32] Renfree, M. 1993. *Ontogeny, genetic control, and phylogeny of female reproduction in monotreme and therian mammals.*

[33] R. M. Nowak. 1991. *Walker's Mammals of the World.* Maryland, Johns Hopkins University Press (edited volume) II [A. Behrensmeyer/A.

[34] Shapiro E, Lepor H, Jeffs RD. The inheritance of the exstrophy-epispadias complex. *J Urol.* 1984 Aug;132(2):308-10.

[35] Hendren WH. Cloacal malformations: experience with 105 cases. *J Pediatr Surg.* 1992 Jul;27(7):890-901.

[36] Hendren WH. Urogenital sinus and cloacal malformations. *Semin Pediatr Surg.* 1996 Feb;5(1):72-9.

[37] Hendren WH. Cloaca, the most severe degree of imperforate anus: experience with 195 cases. *Ann Surg.* 1998 Sep;228(3):331-46.

[38] Levitt MA, Pena A. Pitfalls in the management of newborn cloacas. *Pediatr Surg Int.* 2005 Apr;21(4):264-9.

[39] Yamada G, Suzuki K, Haraguchi R, Miyagawa S, Satoh Y, Kamimura M, et al.. Molecular genetic cascades for external genitalia formation: an emerging organogenesis program. *Dev Dyn.* 2006 Jul;235(7):1738-52.

[40] van der Putte SC. The devlopment of the perineum in the human. A comprehensive histological study with a special reference to the role of the stromal components. *Adv Anat Embryol Cell Biol.* 2005;177:1-131.

[41] van der Putte SC. Normal and abnormal development of the anorectum. *J Pediatr Surg.* 1986 May;21(5):434-40.

[42] Kluth D, Hillen M, Lambrecht W. The principles of normal and abnormal hindgut development. *J Pediatr Surg.* 1995 Aug;30(8):1143-7.

[43] Marker PC, Donjacour AA, Dahiya R, Cunha GR. Hormonal, cellular, and molecular control of prostatic development. *Dev Biol.* 2003 Jan 15;253(2):165-74.

[44] Danforth CH. 1930. Developmental anomalies in a special strain of mice *Am J Anat* 45(2):275-87.

[45] Kluth D, Lambrecht W, Reich P, Buhrer C. SD-mice--an animal model for complex anorectal malformations. *Eur J Pediatr Surg.* 1991 Jun;1(3):183-8.

[46] Mo R, Kim JH, Zhang J, Chiang C, Hui CC, Kim PC. Anorectal malformations caused by defects in sonic hedgehog signaling. *Am J Pathol.* 2001 Aug;159(2):765-74.

[47] Mortlock DP, Post LC, Innis JW. The molecular basis of hypodactyly (Hd): a deletion in Hoxa 13 leads to arrest of digital arch formation. Nat Genet. 1996 Jul;13(3):284-9.

[48] Mortlock DP, Innis JW. Mutation of HOXA13 in hand-foot-genital syndrome. *Nat Genet.* 1997Feb;15(2):179-80.

[49] Goodman FR, Bacchelli C, Brady AF, Brueton LA, Fryns JP, Mortlock DP, et al.. Novel HOXA13 mutations and the phenotypic spectrum of hand-foot-genital syndrome. *Am J Hum Genet.* 2000 Jul;67(1):197-202.

[50] Tuzel E, Samli H, Kuru I, Turkmen S, Demir Y, Maralcan G, et al.. Association of hypospadias with hypoplastic synpolydactyly and role of HOXD13 gene mutations. *Urology.* 2007 Jul;70(1):161-4.

[51] Johnson KR, Sweet HO, Donahue LR, Ward-Bailey P, Bronson RT, Davisson MT. A new spontaneous mouse mutation of Hoxd13 with a polyalanine expansion and phenotype similar to human synpolydactyly. *Hum Mol Genet.* 1998 Jun;7(6):1033-8.

[52] Kondo T, Dolle P, Zakany J, Duboule D. Function of posterior HoxD genes in the morphogenesis of the anal sphincter. *Development.* 1996 Sep;122(9):2651-9.

[53] Ross AJ, Ruiz-Perez V, Wang Y, Hagan DM, Scherer S, Lynch SA, et al.. A homeobox gene, HLXB9, is the major locus for dominantly inherited sacral agenesis. *Nat Genet.* 1998 Dec;20(4): 358-61.

[54] Kessel M, Gruss P. Homeotic transformations of murine vertebrae and concomitant alteration of Hox codes induced by retinoic acid. *Cell.* 1991 Oct 4;67(1):89-104.

[55] Conlon RA, Rossant J. Exogenous retinoic acid rapidly induces anterior ectopic expression of murine Hox-2 genes in vivo. *Development.* 1992 Oct;116(2):357-68.

[56] Ogino Y, Suzuki K, Haraguchi R, Satoh Y, Dolle P, Yamada G. External genitalia formation: role of fibroblast growth factor, retinoic acid signaling, and distal urethral epithelium. *Ann N Y Acad Sci.* 2001 Dec;948:13-31.

[57] Kraus F, Haenig B, Kispert A. Cloning and expression analysis of the mouse T-box gene tbx20. *Mech Dev.* 2001 Jan;100(1):87-91.

[58] Ohta S, Suzuki K, Tachibana K, Tanaka H, Yamada G. Cessation of gastrulation is mediated by suppression of epithelial-mesenchymal transition at the ventral ectodermal ridge. *Development.* 2007 Dec;134(24):4315-24.

[59] Ohta S, Schoenwolf GC, Yamada G. The cessation of gastrulation: BMP signaling and EMT during and at the end of gastrulation. *Cell Adh Migr.* 2010 Jul-Sep;4(3):440-6.

[60] Zakin L, Reversade B, Kuroda H, Lyons KM, De Robertis EM. Sirenomelia in Bmp7 and Tsg compound mutant mice: requirement for Bmp signaling in the development of ventral posterior mesoderm. *Development.* 2005 May;132(10):2489-99.

[61] Suzuki K, Economides A, Yanagita M, Graf D, Yamada G. New horizons at the caudal embryos: coordinated urogenital/reproductive organ formation by growth factor signaling. *Curr Opin Genet Dev.* 2009 Oct;19(5):491-6.

[62] Gordon KJ, Kirkbride KC, How T, Blobe GC. Bone morphogenetic proteins induce pancreatic cancer cell invasiveness through a Smad1-dependent mechanism that involves matrix metalloproteinase-2. *Carcinogenesis.* 2009 Feb;30(2):238-48.

[63] Winnier G, Blessing M, Labosky PA, Hogan BL. Bone morphogenetic protein-4 is required for mesoderm formation and patterning in the mouse. *Genes Dev.* 1995 Sep 1;9(17):2105-16.

[64] Oishi I, Suzuki H, Onishi N, Takada R, Kani S, Ohkawara B, et al.. The receptor tyrosine kinase Ror2 is involved in non-canonical Wnt5a/JNK signalling pathway. *Genes Cells.* 2003 Jul;8(7): 645-54.

[65] Qian D, Jones C, Rzadzinska A, Mark S, Zhang X, Steel KP, et al.. Wnt5a functions in planar cell polarity regulation in mice. *Dev Biol.* 2007 Jun 1;306(1):121-33.

[66] Cook C, Vezina CM, Allgeier SH, Shaw A, Yu M, Peterson RE, et al.. Noggin is required for normal lobe patterning and ductal budding in the mouse prostate. *Dev Biol.* 2007 Dec 1;312(1): 217-30.

[67] Allgeier SH, Lin TM, Vezina CM, Moore RW, Fritz WA, Chiu SY, et al.. WNT5A selectively inhibits mouse ventral prostate development. *Dev Biol.* 2008 Dec 1;324(1):10-7.

[68] Ciani L, Salinas PC. c-Jun N-terminal kinase (JNK) cooperates with Gsk3beta to regulate Dishevelled-mediated microtubule stability. *BMC Cell Biol.* 2007;8:27.

[69] Podkowa M, Zhao X, Chow CW, Coffey ET, Davis RJ, Attisano L. Microtubule stabilization by bone morphogenetic protein receptor-mediated scaffolding of c-Jun N-terminal kinase promotes dendrite formation. *Mol Cell Biol.* 2010 May;30(9):2241-50.

[70] Pyati UJ, Cooper MS, Davidson AJ, Nechiporuk A, Kimelman D. Sustained Bmp signaling is essential for cloaca development in zebrafish. *Development.* 2006 Jun;133(11):2275-84.

[71] Chen T, Li Q, Xu J, Ding K, Wang Y, Wang W, et al.. Mutation screening of BMP4, BMP7, HOXA4 and HOXB6 genes in Chinese patients with hypospadias. *Eur J Hum Genet.* 2007 Jan; 15(1):23-8.

[72] Beleza-Meireles A, Lundberg F, Lagerstedt K, Zhou X, Omrani D, Frisen L, et al.. FGFR2, FGF8, FGF10 and BMP7 as candidate genes for hypospadias. *Eur J Hum Genet.* 2007 Apr;15(4):405-10.

[73] Yamada G, Satoh Y, Baskin LS, Cunha GR. Cellular and molecular mechanisms of development of the external genitalia. *Differentiation.* 2003 Oct;71(8):445-60.

[74] Karner C, Wharton KA, Jr., Carroll TJ. Planar cell polarity and vertebrate organogenesis. *Semin Cell Dev Biol.* 2006 Apr;17(2):194-203.

[75] Song MR, Shirasaki R, Cai CL, Ruiz EC, Evans SM, Lee SK, et al.. T-Box transcription factor Tbx20 regulates a genetic program for cranial motor neuron cell body migration. *Development.* 2006 Dec;133(24):4945-55.

[76] Cayuso J, Ulloa F, Cox B, Briscoe J, Marti E. The Sonic hedgehog pathway independently controls the patterning, proliferation and survival of neuroepithelial cells by regulating Gli activity. *Development.* 2006 Feb;133(3):517-28.

In: Handbook of Genitourinary Medicine: New Research   ISBN: 978-1-62618-226-4
Editor: Rashmi R. Singh   © 2013 Nova Science Publishers, Inc.

Chapter VI

From Bench to Patients: Advances in Genitourinary Regenerative Medicine

S. Bouhout[1]*, A. Rousseau[1]*, F. Bouchard[2],* A. Morissette[1], S. Chabaud[1] and S. Bolduc[1,2]

[1]Laboratoire d'Organogenèse Expérimentale/LOEX, Centre de recherche FRQS du CHU de Québec, Medicine Faculty, Laval University, Quebec City, Quebec, Canada
[2]Department of Surgery, CHUQ, Laval University, Quebec City, Quebec, Canada

Abstract

Tissue engineering is an emerging field which could be the answer to many medical issues, notably when tissue or organ, native or artificial, are not available in sufficient quantities or quality, or to solve ethical problem when animal experimentation could be replace by a near in-vivo environment.

Such a problem exists in genitourinary medicine when there is a need for augmentation or replacement of genitourinary tissues: the specificity of these tissues, bladder, urethra or vagina for example, does not allow the use of other tissue without the risk of potential severe complications for the patients. Replacement tissues should mimic the features of the healthy native one. In the case of genitourinary tissues, their specific characteristics are mainly attributed to the epithelium. They also must grow and differentiate appropriately. So far, several solutions have been proposed based on already prepared scaffolds: biomaterials, such as PGA family members, or acellular tissues, such as small intestinal submucosa (SIS), or the bladder acellular matrix graft (BAMG).

All these tissue engineering techniques have their strengths and weaknesses. Graft rejection or inappropriate differentiation and/or organization of epithelial cells all remain a challenge, particularly in the case of a large scale application of these techniques.

---

* Authors contributed equally.

Another crucial problem which must be taken into account in paediatric genitourinary medicine: the graft has to grow with the patient. For now, we do not have a sufficient retrospect to be sure, not only of the long term safeness of the implant, but also of the ability of this graft to co-evolve with the patients. To limit the discomforts for the patients and health cost related to theses pathologies, it could be recommended to adopt safer and more sustainable solutions. An alternative strategy, proposed by Dr Bolduc's *laboratoire d'organogenèse expérimentale des tissues urologiques* (LOETU), could be the use of self-assembled engineered tissues. Contrarily to other techniques used in tissue engineering, the self-assembly approach is free of exogenous material. In this technique, the cells themselves produce their own extracellular matrix, which creates a near in-vivo cell environment. It has been shown that these stromas can reproduce not only healthy and pathologic environments but also change the fate of the on-top seeded epithelium. Autologous equivalents have already been produced for pigs (bladder) and humans (urethra and bladder). Urethral and vaginal tissues for rabbit models are in the phase of optimisation.

The purpose of this article is to present a history of the use of tissue engineering in genitourinary regenerative medicine, to review the existing methods at the moment and to point toward perspectives for surgical treatments and the potential development of more ethical and more accurate in vitro models for studies.

1. Introduction: Anatomy and Pathology of Genitourinary Tissues

Urinary system is essential in itself: it filters the blood from its wastes, maintains electrolytic homeostasis and water balance. It consists of several organs and tissues (Figure 1): the kidneys which filter the blood and condensate urine, the ureters which carry this latter liquid to the bladder, the bladder which is responsible of the storage of urine between two micturitions, and the urethra which allows evacuation of urine during urination. All the excretory system has to be impermeable, so that the urine can not diffuse into bloodstream. For the purpose of this chapter, only the lower urinary tract, bladder and urethra, will be studied.

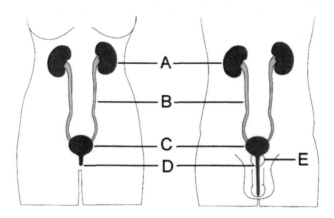

Figure 1. Urinary systems in women and men.A) Kidneys. B) Ureters. C) Bladder. D) Urethra. Please note the similarity of both systems except for the urethra.

Genital organs are responsible of reproductive function. They are obviously different for males and females even if several similarities could be found. In this chapter, we focus only on the urethra and the vagina.

1.1. Bladder

Bladder is a temporary urine reservoir. Watertightness and compliance are its two main features. Complex mechanisms, involving nervous system, allow the filling and emptying of the bladder with urine [1]. Bladder must accommodate various volume of liquid without an increase of pressure which could be damageable to the kidneys [2]. This role is mainly due to the detrusor, the bladder muscle [1]. Bladder must also be a safe storage for the toxic components of urine such as urea. This is the role of bladder sphincter and urothelium, the bladder epithelium [3].

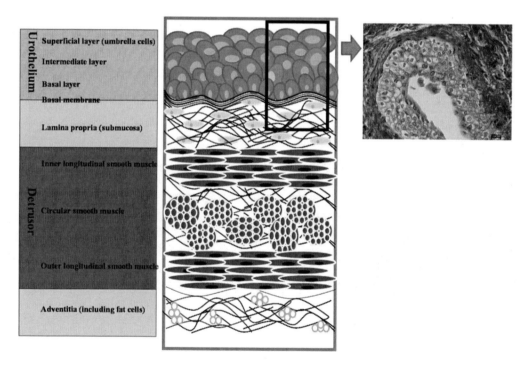

Figure 2. Bladder anatomy. Bladder anatomy is depicted in the left and central panels. A Masson's trichrome staining of slice from a rabbit bladder is presented in the right panel.

Briefly, the bladder consists in four distinct layers (Figure 2). From the exterior of the organ to the interior, we found first the adventitia, the muscular layer, the submucosa layer and, finally, the urothelium [4]. The adventitia is a connective tissue layer vascularized and innervated. The nerves participate to coordinate the emptying of the bladder. Some adipose tissue could also be founded in this layer. Muscles are organized in three sub layers separated by spans of connective tissue: the outer layer of longitudinal muscle fibres, a layer of circular muscle fibres, and the inner layer of longitudinal muscle fibres. This muscle allows the contraction of the bladder to expulse urine during urination. Presence of elastic fibres allows the compliance of the bladder and maintains a low-pressure reservoir during the filling. The submucosa is a connective tissue joining the detrusor and the urothelium. The role of this layer is very important in order to maintain a well organized and functional epithelium. The extracellular matrix is not only a support tissue but is also involved in signalling. It could be further a reserve from growth factors and cytokines [5].

This tissue is mainly constituted of collagen type I and III fibres [6, 7], elastic fibres and unmyelinated nervous endings [8]. Microcapillaries allow the feeding of the epithelial layer. Finally the urothelium lays on a coating of very specific extracellular matrix proteins such as laminin and collagen IV called basal lamina. The bladder epithelium [3] is a pseudostratified one; all the urothelial cells are attached on the basal lamina. It mainly consists in three sub layers. First, the basal cells, containing cubic cells, are the progenitors [9] and very low differentiated cells [10]. Then, the intermediate cells, organized in various number of levels depending on the filling status of the bladder. They begin their differentiation, and, at the more internal level, the superficial cells can be found. They are called umbrella cells and are the most differentiated type of urothelial cells [11, 12]. Umbrella cells organize at their surface a protein complex specific to the urothelium, the uroplakin plaque, which is the terminal marker of urothelial differentiation. Tight junctions between cells and uroplakins assure the impermeability of the bladder [13-16].

Pathologies and Surgical Reconstruction

The main necessities for surgical reconstruction of the bladder are congenital malformations such as vesical extrophy, neurogenic bladders, which result from congenital defects but also from acquired diseases such as diabetes or trauma, bladder cancers, mostly caused by tobacco, and several other problems.

Life quality is severely compromised by the loss of function of this organ. This is why all of these pathologies could require augmentation or replacement of the urinary bladder. At the moment, after numerous trials using urologic or non urologic tissues [17-20], the gold standard technique for surgical bladder repair or reconstruction is the use of intestinal segment [21]. The choice of the segment depends mainly on age and medical history. Nevertheless, the surgical procedure in itself and the obvious different biological functions of the intestine and the bladder, often leads to complications [22, 23] such as intestinal occlusion, hypocontractility, hematuria, dysuria, urolithiasis, neoplasia, ectopic mucus production and metabolic imbalances due to urine absorption by the intestinal mucosa, which can induce delay of growth and reduction of bone density in pediatric patients [24-29].

1.2. Urethra

When the bladder is filled, the urine must be evacuated outside of the organism. The coordination of muscle contraction and sphincters relaxation allows the liquid to pass through the urethra [1]. The urethra is a tubular structure composed of multiple layers of tissues [4]. The structure of the tube is roughly similar to the one of the bladder: smooth muscles with intra-fascicular connective tissue, submucosa or lamina propria with collagen fibres and microvascularization, and finally, the urethral epithelium lays on the basal lamina. The male urethra presents the same features of the bladder urothelium in its proximal part (prostatic urethral segment) contrary to its lower part. After the prostatic segment of urethra (about four centimetres), the epithelium becomes cylindrical and stratified when it passes through the perineum (about one centimetre). Prostatic and perineal segments also present a thick longitudinal muscular inner layer and a thin circular muscular outer layer. In the last part of urethra (fifteen centimetres), epithelium is also cylindrical but bistratified. Female urethra is most simple with only two parts in its three centimetres. The first proximal third is roughly similar to the male one but the two distal thirds are comparable to the epidermis with a pluristratified epithelium.

Pathologies and Surgical Reconstruction

Several pathologies can affect urethra [30]. They usually are classified in two major groups: the congenital urethral pathologies and the acquired ones. For example, in the first group there are urethral diverticulum, lack of penis, micropenis, hypospadias, epispadias [31] and double urethra. In the second group, urethral strictures, fistulaes and cancers can be found. In the case of epispadia, where urethra ends in an inappropriate dorsal location on the penis, the bladder is also often affected. Several steps of reconstruction can be necessary. Hypospadias, where the urethral end is on the ventral side of the penis, also needs complex reconstructive surgeries.

For now, patients are treated with autologous graft of penile skin or foreskin [32]. Some complications are observed like contraction, fistulae, stenosis, ectopic hairs, etc... Oral mucosas are also used with similar troubles [33].

1.3. Vagina

In Humans

In a histological point of view [4], the vagina is a muscular membranous tube consisting of four different layers. The most external layer, called adventitia, represents the periphery of the organ. It consists of connective tissue and some adipose cells. The second layer includes the beams of smooth muscle fibres. These fibres can be grouped in two categories: the internal circular layer and the longitudinal external one. These muscular layers may contract during sexual intercourse. The third section, the lamina propria /submucosa, contains the major part of the blood vessels of the vagina as well as an important lymphatic network. This layer is devoid of gland and the vagina is lubricated by cervical mucus and mucus from glands in the labia minora. Extracellular matrix of this chorion consists mainly of elastic and collagen fibres. Finally, the epithelium, or mucosa, is pavimentous, stratified, squamous and non-keratinized. The vaginal epithelial cells are rather round at the level of the basal membrane, where there are mitoses, and the more they move towards the lumen, the more they become more flattened and their nuclei condense until cells die and are removed from the tissue by desquamation.

In Rabbits

In the rabbit, the cellular and matrix composition of the vagina is roughly the same as the human one [34] except at the level of the vaginal epithelium [35]. Indeed, this last one consists of only one or two layers (Figure 3) of cubic and cylindrical cells, rather than to be stratified pavimentous like it is in human. This difference supports the hypothesis that the vaginal epitheliums from the two species could have slightly different functions.

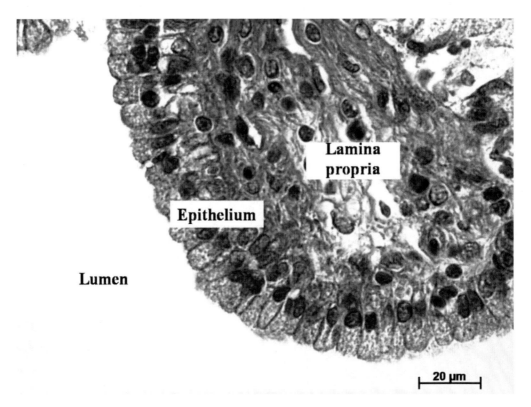

Figure 3. Histology from a rabbit vagina. Masson's trichrome staining from a slice of a rabbit vagina. Note the bistratified vaginal epithelium.

Pathologies and Surgical Reconstruction

Vulvovaginal reconstruction procedures have been practised for many years. Among pathologies affecting the vagina is the vaginal agenesis, usually as Mayer-Robitansky-Kuster-Hauser (MRKH) syndrome (1 per 4000 female) [36]. This syndrome is defined as congenital absence of the vagina, with primary amenorrhea and normal secondary sexual characteristics. The external genitalia seem normal and the uterine /gonadal development is variable. Furthermore, vulvovaginal reconstruction is also indicated in cases of cloacal exstrophy, bladder exstrophy and urogenital sinus malformations, oncologic exanteration and transsexuals male-to-female surgeries.

No perfect tissue for such surgeries has been found yet. Usage of skin grafts (often using Abbè-McIndoe technique) [37], buccal mucosa grafts [38], amniotic membranes, myocutaneous flaps [39], bowel transplantation with colon or ileum [40-42], peritoneum and allogeneic tissues have all been tempted, with acceptable results. Limitations to grafting techniques are often the small quantity of accessible tissue, scars and pain. Furthermore, the implanted tissue is obviously non-reactive to hormonal stimulation, often predisposes to infections, sometimes causes foul smelling odours or mucoid secretion, [36, 42], and usage of lubricants for sexual usage is necessary. Strictures or stenosis on short and long-term follow-up are another complication sometimes reported [42]. Thus, the need for stenting is mandatory in most techniques used, and the achievement of a functional vagina takes months to years, sometimes needing long term dilator use. Non-invasive techniques such as dilator use only without surgery also represent a successful approach in some very motivated patient suffering MRKH syndrome [41]. The classic Abbè-McIndoe technique [37, 43] consists of a skin graft being implanted in the neovaginal space. Normal vaginal mucosa progressively replaces the graft, but it is unknown if it is simply due to extension from normal vaginal vestibule tissue or metaplasia from the skin graft. Some teams have, in recent years, tempted to reproduce the tissue engineering techniques known so far to create a neovaginal tissue using autologous tissue. Potential advantages are reduced operative times, better postoperative evolution (less complications), better long term success, no rejection, diminished risk of infectious disease transmission, a potential positive psychological role, absence of dyspareunia or mucous discharge. Interesting experiences and results have been published yet, which will be reviewed later.

1.4. Importance of Epithelial Differentiation

Due to its toxicity, the urine must not disseminate in the body. The watertightness function of urologic tissues is mainly afforded by the epithelium and notably the bladder urothelium, because it is for longer times in contact with the urine during its storage. This feature can only be properly achieved with a well differentiation of the superficial cells, the umbrella cells. Tightness of junctions between cells and presence of a mature uroplakin plaques are the better markers of this status. Tissues used to date do not present these characteristics and then could not support for optimal vesical reconstruction. For other genitourinary tissues, it is clear that the more the epithelium is similar in nature to the native one, the more it could play the same role than the native tissue and the more the epithelium could play these roles, the more the near native functions will be established.

2. History of Tissue Engineering in Genitourinary Reconstructive Medicine

2.1. Synthetic Scaffold

Synthetic polymers are biomaterials made of macromolecules assembled with covalent links. Depending on their physical properties, they are classified in three groups: thermoplastics, thermo-hardenings and elastomers. The main advantage of synthetic polymers is the capacity to manufacture any forms of organ in three-dimensions, in a quantitative and reproducible way, at relatively low cost. Because it is an artificial material, it eliminates the problems related to tissue harvesting. Moreover many characteristics can be controlled such as porosity and mechanical properties. These biomaterials are degraded by hydrolysis and fragments removed through metabolic pathways [44-46]. The molecular weight and copolymerisation ratio are factors which determine the degradation rate of synthetic materials. The challenge for this synthetic scaffold is to provide an ideal microenvironment for cell-matrix and cell-cell communications. It has been proved that synthetic materials enhance adherence, growth and migration of seeded cells [47]. How they can manage differentiation into a well organized tissue remains a challenge. This last cellular event could be dictated by several physical and biochemical properties which can be specifically modulated. For transplantation, the optimal synthetic scaffold must have a controlled degradation. It must remain stable until the recruitment and infiltration of the surrounding cells, but must not persist and jeopardize the neo-tissue regeneration. Pore size is another significant parameter. Scale of size pores modulates cellular migration, vascular invasion, and diffusion of nutrients, waste and oxygen [48, 49].

2.2. Decellularised Matrices

This type of substitute is prepared from native tissue which is decellularised, and then sterilised with numerous methods [50]. The general principle consists of discarding cells with physical, enzymatic or chemical protocols [51]. This model presents a mechanical and biochemical environment ideal for the cellular recognition. This is a considerable advantage because it is known that extracellular matrix guides the cells to the organ development, repair and regeneration. The extracellular matrix proteins and their physiological organization can induce a suitable signalling to cells and allow their migration and proliferation through the scaffold [52]. But chemicals treatments for the decellularisation and sterilisation are often aggressive towards extracellular matrix proteins [53]. Indeed, biophysical elements like the increase of temperature and pH, or biochemical agents like ionic detergents denature these proteins which become unfolded. Thus, the extracellular matrix architecture is disrupted and mechanicals properties, as elasticity or resistance, are lost [54]. On another hand, the use of decellularised matrices as support for cellular proliferation and differentiation is interesting because of its composition in growth factors. But their removal can be caused by the sterilisation process such as chemicals treatments, dry heat and pressurized steam [53]. In this domain, the use of paracetic acid submersion has been a progress to preserve some of the growth factors [55, 56]. Another quality of this type of substitute is the ability to support the neovascularization after transplantation which is important to provide a nutritive supply and to promote the graft survival [57, 58].

2.3. Bladder

Polyglycolic acid (PGA) and polylactic-co-glycolic acid (PLGA) have been primarily used for bladder scaffold confection. They are attractive because it is easy to control the ratio of lactide: glycolide and molecular weight. Like decellularised tissues, studies revealed the importance of seeding polymer scaffolds with urologic cells. *In vivo*, PGA/PLGA scaffolds without cell seeded underwent shrinkage after one month post-graft [59]. On the other hand, when urothelial cells are seeded on the luminal surface and smooth muscle cells are seeded on the opposite side, the synthetic construct is capable to retain urine at short-term. However, in spite of this relative success, the synthetic substitute is devoid of inherent biological activity and the cells distribution seems to be concentrated at the periphery rather than in a homogeneous way. At long term, clinical tests were performed on patient suffering from pathological non-compliant bladder, and candidates for cystoplasty [60]. The synthetic substitute was seeded with urothelial and smooth muscle cells, and placed in vivo for bladder repair. Several elements had to be taken into account. Firstly, to promote the cellular recognition and adherence, collagen was added to the PGA scaffold. Secondly, the synthetic scaffold was wrapped with the highly vascularized omentum in order to support the graft survival. Unfortunately, positive results have been assessed only for one of the seven patients. The urological cells showed a proper distribution but the bladder compliance has not been generalized for all of patients. To optimize the cellular development, synthetic peptides derived from extracellular matrix protein could be incorporated within scaffolds: e.g. RGD sequence, a cell adhesive, integrin-binding peptide found in fibronectin and laminin [61].

Two types of tissue are decellularised in order to repair a defected bladder. The small intestinal submucosa (SIS) was the first to be considered because of its rich composition in glycoaminoglycans, glycoproteins and various types of collagen (type I, III and IV). These structural proteins form an extracellular matrix with a suitable architecture for the storage of growth factors. The heparan sulfate proteoglycans (HSPG), fibroblast growth factor 2 (FGF2), transforming growth factor beta (TGF-β), and the vascular endothelial growth factor (VEGF) have been detected in decellularised SIS [62], which is preferable to the cellular growth, as well as to promote the graft neovascularization. Decellularised SIS have been marketed and used for bladder reconstruction. However a lot of postoperative inflammations have been described [63] and, *in vitro*, DNA residues have been detected [64], which implicate the decellularisation process efficiency. In animal models, decellularised SIS have been used to ameliorate the bladder capacity. After the seeding of urothelial and smooth muscle cells [65], a suitable adherence was observed onto the decellularised SIS, but their differentiation were not induced. Transplantation in four dogs has been realised and led to a limited success [66]. The compliance was improved during 9 months post-operative, but one of fourth died because of a perforation within the SIS graft. The unsuitable differentiation of seeded urothelial cells could explain this fact, because without their watertight function urine can denature extracellular matrix proteins and destroy the matrix architecture.

The lack of a good cellular organization could be logically assigned to the lack of conform protein-cell signalling, because the SIS and bladder extracellular matrix are different [67]. Thus, researches have focused toward the use of decellularised bladder, named bladder acellular matrix graft (BAMG). The interest of this model is based on the fact that urothelial cell behavior is obviously affected by the extracellular matrix, which is present within the *lamina propria* [68]. However, even if the nature of the BAMG scaffold appeared more conform for bladder cell development, compared to the SIS, the limitations due to the decellularisation process remain the same. It has been shown that the BAMG preparation permits the collagen type I and laminin preservation, while fibronectin and laminin which are principal components of basal lamina are altered [69]. All cellular layers of the urothelium are directly in contact with the basal lamina, and a failure cell signalling through matrix proteins could compromise the *in vitro* regeneration of a bladder substitute. Implantation of a seeded BAMG in a porcine model demonstrated bladder cell infiltration which remained limited to the periphery of the substitute [70]. The insufficient cellular organization resulted in calcification formation within the graft and its shrinkage. Beyond the aspect of matrix support, the tissue culture techniques have to be taken into account. The bladder is subjected to different pressures during the emptying/filling cycle, therefore a bioreactor capable of delivering hydrostatic pressure waves has been developed and tested with urothelial and smooth muscle cells seeded on BAMG model [71]. The expression of matrix proteins increased and could constitute an alternative to the damage caused by the decellularisation protocol. Dynamic culture provides other positive results, like the increase of expression of uroplakin II, a specific marker of urothelial differentiation.

2.4. Urethra

The principal advantage of using a synthetic polymer is that it eliminates the risk of stone encrustation or hair in the urethral lumen that can be found with the hair baring skin. In 1992, a combination of polyhydroxybutyric acid (PHB) and PGA was used to elaborate a urethral substitute [72]. An urethroplasty was performed on a dog model and the synthetic scaffold has been resorbed after 8 months. Histological results showed the conservation of lumen. In 1997, a scaffold made of hyaluronan benzyl ester (Hyaff-11) was used on a rabbit model at short-term [73]. This material was chosen for its wound healing potential, but microfistulas were observed at the suture site. PGA and PLGA were also used for urethral reconstruction. This type of substitute was seeded with bovine chondrocytes because of the ability to implant these cells in the genitourinary tract has been demonstrated for many urological treatments [74-76]. The biocompatibility has been established and this model supported the urine contact. Poly L-polylactic acid (PLLA) is another polymer used to construct a stent seeded with urothelial cells from the urethra [77]. Its mechanical properties offer the possibility to avoid urethral collapse. Good cellular adherence was obtained and the synthetic scaffold was degraded after 12 weeks. Finally, rabbit represents the best animal model for urethral repair, and diverse biomaterial scaffolds demonstrated good results, but no long-term study has been completed so far.

SIS and BAMG were also used for urethral reconstruction. A porcine SIS was used for a rabbit urethroplasty during three months [78]. The feasibility was established, but the short-term character of this intervention does not permit to evaluate the efficiency of this method. BAMG was also tested because of its common endodermal origin with urethra, which could lead to a suitable integration of the graft. Also it is easily prepared and conserved until its use [79, 80]. Some studies had reported the confection of porcine BAMG into tubular shape for urethral repair [81]. This substitute was used during 1 month on a rabbit model and demonstrated the importance of the cells seeding onto the scaffold. Indeed, unseeded BAMG scaffold shows efficiency for a urethral repair requiring a substitute for less than 0.5 centimetre. But, over 1 centimetre, the study recommended the presence of cells in order to improve the graft remodelling and avoid stricture at term. Another study underlines the importance to use urologic cells for urologic defects [82]. For example, oral epithelial cells was seeded onto BAMG, showing a good biocompatibility and confirming the presence of seeded scaffold rather than unseeded [83, 84]. But these oral keratinocytes organized themselves onto squamous stratified epithelium, whereas urothelium is transitional pseudo-stratified. Decellularised aortic matrix has also been tested as experimental model for urethral defect [85]. The tubular form and the good mechanical properties made it a model of choice. Until now, good results were obtained but no long-term evaluation has been performed. Finally, decellularised urethra was also used for its extracellular matrix proteins and cytokines composition and localization. Rabbit urethroplasty was made with allogeneic acellular urethral matrix for 6 months, but their results showed a partial success from a functional and histological point of view [86].

2.5. Vagina

Inert materials have also been used for vaginal reconstruction, such as artificial dermis, collagen sponges or decellularized matrix, showing subsequent epithelisation.

Vaginal Epithelial Cell Culture

Vaginal epithelial cell culture has to be successful prior to thinking of bioengineering a neotissue. In 1959, a team evaluated the vaginal response of rats in vivo to oestrogen exposure. The cornification process of the epithelium was related with the dose of oestrogen. This work demonstrated a clear effect of the hormone on this epithelium in vivo [87]. Also in 1959, Kahn showed that vitamin A, a precursor of retinoic acid, seemed to prevent or delay vaginal epithelial cells keratinization in vitro, while B-oestradiol seemed to accelerate it [88]. Later, in 1979, Kaye, Sobel, Tchao et al.. made 2mm cubes of vaginal epithelium and put them in a culture medium including amphotericin B. They obtained multilayered growth at 2-3 weeks, then, colony stopped growing. Rare fibroblast contaminations were seen on gross examination. Formation of squames occurred at the fourth week as seen in vivo. They showed marked difference between upper and bottom-most layer of cells, like tonofilaments, mitochondria and endoplasmic reticulum abundance. Keratinization and desquamation of the superficial cells, similar to normal exfoliated cells, suggested retention of the in vivo phenotype, according to themselves [89]. In 1986-7, a team evaluated seeded vaginal epithelial cells of mice on collagen gels and on plastics (unpublished results for plastics because no growth). They tried many different combinations, at first showing better proliferative potential with full serum free Dulbecco's Modified Eagle's Ham (DH) medium supplemented with insulin, EGF, Cholera toxin, transferrin and bovine serum albumin fraction V (BSA). Surprisingly, the proliferative potential was diminished when using bovine serum, and was dose responsive with horse serum. The most important of all the additives tested was clearly insulin, which showed great proliferative action. The cumulative effect of the additives was also seen when each medium was tested with only one of the additives. This experience showed no effect from any of the additive when used alone in serum free DH, except insulin. No hormonal effects on proliferation with progesterone or 17B-oestradiol (E2) were seen, but rather an inhibitory effect when increasing concentration. They also tested medium with and without phenol red, considering the low oestrogenic effect known of this agent, showing no difference. They concluded hypothesising the serum could contain an inhibitor of estrogen target cell proliferation [90, 91]. They also described the inhibitory effect of E2 in a subsequent experience. Then, because the absence or low quantity of oestrogen receptor (ER) was thought as another potential cause for unresponsiveness to hormones, they extracted the cells differently, using the Percoll density gradient [92, 93] centrifugation for separating epithelial cells from stromal cells and cellular debris, which is supposed to better preserve the steroid receptors. As E2 still inhibited cell proliferation, many hypotheses were still proposed like an insulin effect on cytosolic ER concentration. Are there paracrine factors that are absent because the cells are not grown on a vaginal stroma [94]? In a subsequent paper, they showed clear E2 response of vaginal stroma and uterine stroma culture, but at different concentration (10 -12 M and 10 -8 M). In 1989, another team grew ecto and endocervical epithelial cells in vitro with no fibroblast feeder layer. They characterised effectively the ectocervical (vaginal) cells positive for keratin 13 and cells had the squamous epithelial morphology [95]. In 1990, a team described an extraction technique for vaginal epithelial cells. They grew the cells on a collagen sponge matrix and on plastic, showing a better cohesion between cells while grown on collagen. They had hexagonal shape and were flat, then formed multilayer at day 21.

The epithelium had a slightly slower growth rate in collagen compared to plastic (15 days), but had a better potential for structural arrangement [96]. In 2007 and 2009, Zong et al.. [97, 98] analysed the matrix composition of human vaginal fibroblasts cultured with different concentration of progesterone and oestrogen. They showed that the Matrix Metalloproteinase (MMP) 1 and 13 were clearly regulated by the presence of the sexual steroids. There were more pro-MMP but less active form in the case of hormone stimulated tissues compared to control.

Tissue Engineering Reconstruction of Vagina

In 2007, an Italian team [99] reported a single case of vaginoplasty using autologous in vitro cultured vaginal tissue in a MRKH patient. They extracted epithelial cells from a vaginal biopsy. These cells were then seeded onto four collagen IV-coated culture plates. They were maintained in MCDB-153 medium for 2 weeks. These were then mounted on 2mg/10cm2 hyaluronic acid embedded gauze, and finally implanted successfully in the patient. In 2009, a team seeded vaginal epithelial cells on type 1 collagen-coated dextran microcarrier beads. They grew the tissue in a rotating bioreactor and showed better differentiation than same epithelial cells cultures in a monolayer in 2D. They used their model to test new microbicides for potential toxicity and efficiency in prevention of sexual transmitted diseases (STD) [100]. In 2009, Zhao et al.. [38] reported the mouth autologous micromucosa graft for vaginoplasty in 9 patients. They proved success in most of their interventions.

Long-term results are yet to be known. In 2010, Stany et al.. [39] reported the usage of an acellular dermal allograft, processed from a human cadaver. It obviates the need for allogeneic tissue. One patient out of 4 had agglutination of the neovagina. In 2011, Dorin et al.. [101] reported vaginal reconstruction in rabbits using autologous tissue. They placed several strips of smooth muscle in culture.

At cell confluence, broadly reacting cytokeratin and alpha-actin were used to confirm the phenotype. A polyglycolid acid scaffold was sterilized and the cells were seeded on both sides. They were then cultured for 1 to 7 days before implantation. Cell-seeded scaffolds were implanted subcutaneously in mice, and later on in another experience, neovagina were implanted successfully in rabbits.

3. Alternate Strategy: Self-Assembled Engineered Tissue

The self-assembly method is able to produce a tissue build by the cells themselves i.e. without the use of any neither exogenic nor acellular biologic material. This method utilizes the potential of the cells to create their own matrix and, then, their own environment. Since several years now, this method has been explored for the reconstruction of urologic tissues [102-108].

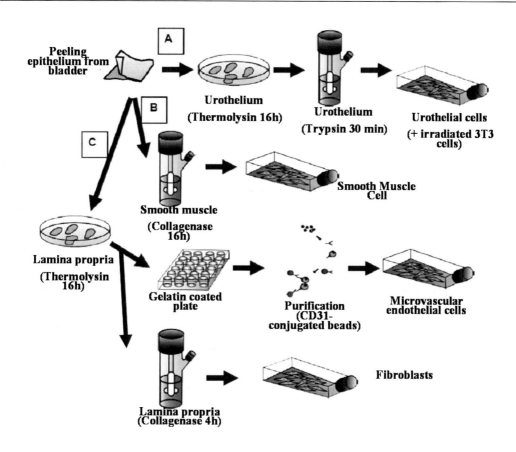

Figure 4. Cell extraction from a bladder biopsy. A) Extraction of urothelial (epithelial) cells. B) Extraction of smooth muscle cells. C) Extraction of microvascular endothelial cells and fibroblasts.

3.1. The self-assembly Technique

Almost all research teams in tissue engineered urologic reconstruction try to work with either synthetic or acelluar biologic matrices. With the evolution of tissue engineering, maybe other paths should be investigated to try to achieve genitourinary tissues. The self-assembly technique is a tissue engineering method developed by LOEX mostly for burn patients. Nevertheless, it proves to be useful for tissue reconstructions ranging from skin to blood vessels [109-111]. In this method, cells, which come from the patient, produce and organize their own extracellular matrix without the use of any neither exogenic nor acellular biologic material. As the cells come from the patient to be transplanted, they are capable of organizing their own microenvironment and limit problem of inflammation and rejection of the graft. This technology is used with impressive results for burned patients since 1986. Organization and composition of extracellular matrix play a very important role in tissue engineering because it has not only a structuring function but also serves as a reservoir of essential factors for the biological functions of the tissues [5]. In the self assembly method, cells receive right signalling for their appropriate differentiation. Physiological [102-104, 110-114] or pathological [115-117] differentiation has been obtained. Then, it results that the transplanted engineered tissue is very similar to the one which have to be replaced.

Cells must be extracted from the patient biopsy (Figure 4). In order to minimize the invasiveness character of this step, several techniques were developed to maximize quantity and purity of cells which could be obtained from a biopsy [106, 109, 118]. Fibroblasts and microvascular endothelial cells can be extracted from dermis or oral mucosa, adipose-derived stromal cells from hypodermis, the fat layer of the skin, smooth muscle cells, vesical fibroblasts, and urothelial cells from bladder or urethra and, finally, smooth muscle cells, vaginal fibroblasts and vaginal epithelial cells from vagina. Briefly, biopsy is submitted to several sequential enzymatic treatments to favour cell-cell or cell-matrix interactions. They are expanded in specific media and on adequate substratum to preserve their phenotypes.

3.2. Bladder

After cell extraction, the bladder substitute can be produced (Figure 5). Stromal cells, whatever their origin, are cultivated in the presence of ascorbate to enhance collagen synthesis, secretion and deposition in order to constitute the extracellular matrix. After three weeks, urothelial cells are seeded onto the top of the stromal component, a preassembled three sheets of fibroblasts. Cells are allowed to proliferate for one week then the equivalent is placed to be cultured at the air/liquid interface for three more weeks.

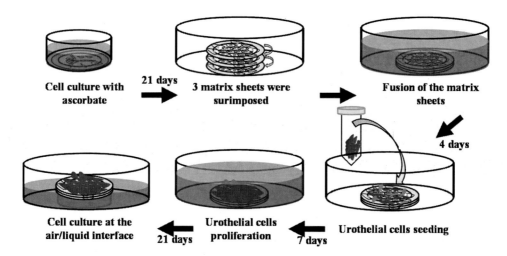

Figure 5. Production of a vesical equivalent by the self assembly technique. Vesical equivalent reconstruction can be divided in two major steps: deposition of extracellular matrix to create a manipulatable sheet followed by proliferation and differentiation of urothelial cells.

As said previously, the combination of tissue engineering and the use of bioreactor (Figure 6) could significantly improve the reconstruction of urologic tissues. By preconditioning the reconstructed tissue in a dynamic environment to simulate the filling and emptying cycles of the bladder, the use of bioreactor may enhance the mechanical behavior of the extracellular matrix [103]. Moreover, it has been demonstrated that a dynamic environment can lead to a better differentiation of the urothelial cell compared to a static one

[104]. The flow and pressure seem to stimulate the expression of not only uroplakin II but also of CK20, two well known terminal markers of the differentiation of the urothelial cells [119].

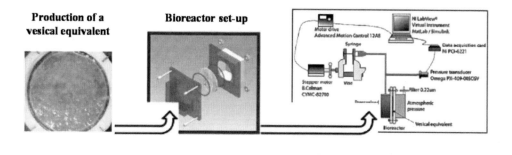

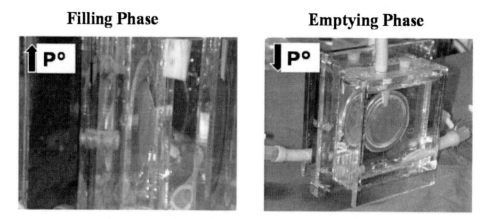

Figure 6. Bioreactor used to enhance urothelial cell differentiation. Bioreactor mimics filling and emptying phases of the bladder. Note that under pressure, vesical equivalent adopts a concave form.

The feasibility of the reconstruction of an autologous human urologic tissue has been demonstrated (Figure 7) but, in order to continue to ameliorate the self-assembly technique adapted to the bladder reconstruction, the use of adipose-derived stromal cells could be investigated. These cells present a particular interest for the tissue engineering due to their great potential. Their capacity to be used to reconstruct skin and adipose tissue equivalents has been already proved [113].

They are fairly easy to obtain and a small biopsy could generate a large number of adipose derived stromal cells [120]. These cells have been described to be able to secrete mediators which are essential to the endothelial cell culture and then vascularization of the graft such as vascular endothelial growth factor (VEGF), hepatocyte growth factor (HGF), fibroblast growth factor (FGF) and the stromal-cell derived factor-1 (SDF-1) [121]. SDF-1 is a mediator that could be linked to the formation of new capillaries by attracting endothelial cells [122].

The angiogenesis is a key factor for the graft take. This complex process allows the supply of the graft with nutriment and oxygen, then reducing necrotic and apoptotic fates of transplanted cells [123, 124].

Additionally, these cells have shown the potential to decrease immune response of Th2 in a respiratory model. Even after an activation of the immune response by TNF-α, the conditioning medium of the adipose derived stromal cells had an anti-inflammatory effect over U937 cells [124, 125].

A sub-population of stem cell exists in the adipose-derived stromal cell populations and is evaluated around 2% of the total cells. These cells add plasticity to the self-assembly model and, in a very interesting manner, adipose-derives stem cells could differentiate mostly in smooth muscle cells after transplantation. All those advantages need to be investigated further and they could be crucial for the graft take and function of a reconstructed tissue.

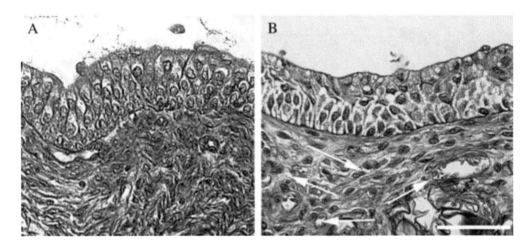

Figure 7. Self Assembly technique allows production of human reconstructed endothelialized vesical equivalent. Left panel: Masson's trichrome staining of a slice from a native porcine bladder. Right panel: Masson's trichrome staining of a slice from a human reconstructed endothelialized vesical equivalent. Note the presence of numerous capillary structures in the tissue (white arrows).

Pig Urinary Bladder Equivalent Reconstruction

Experiments have to be done in animals before clinical translation to humans. In the case of the bladder, pig is an appropriate model. Nevertheless, the self-assembly method was designed to reconstruct the stromal compartment from human fibroblasts. Even if the in-vitro cell culture of fibroblasts from the two species give pretty similar results concerning adhesion and proliferation, it does not seem to work in the same way for the self-assembly of the extracellular matrix.

Optimisation of the protocols has been necessary. Several parameters must be changed to achieve a good matrix deposition. Between the various stromal cells available, fibroblasts from the pig oral mucosa seemed to be the most suitable for the self-assembly method (Figure 8). Furthermore, the temperature seems to play a key role in the deposition of the collagen produced by the porcine fibroblasts.

As internal temperature of pigs is 39°C, if the fibroblasts from the oral mucosa are cultured in this condition the production of the matrix is increased in an acceptable manner [108]. It is interesting to note that fibroblasts from human skin can produce a handable matrix sheet as well at 37°C as 39°C (unpublished Chabaud S. data).

Human reconstructed dermis   **Porcine reconstructed oral mucosa**

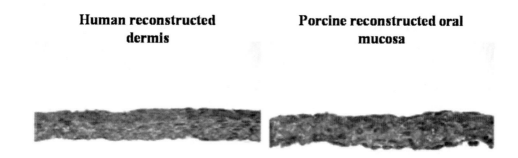

Figure 8. Production of a porcine oral mucosal stroma. Left panel: Masson's trichrome staining of a slice from a human reconstructed dermis. Right panel: Masson's trichrome staining of a slice from a porcine reconstructed oral mucosal stroma.

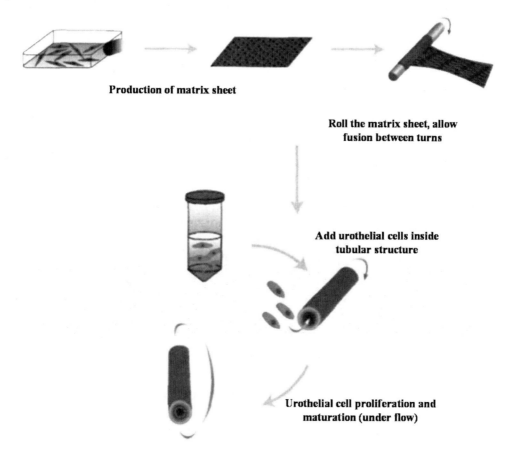

Production of matrix sheet

Roll the matrix sheet, allow fusion between turns

Add urothelial cells inside tubular structure

Urothelial cell proliferation and maturation (under flow)

From Larouche, D. and Ouellet, G. (LOEX)

Figure 9. Production of a tubular urethral equivalent. After a first step of production of a matrix sheet by fibroblasts, the second step is the rolling of the sheet to form a tube. Third, urothelial cells are seeded and differentiate under flow.

3.3. Urethra

In Humans

Tissue engineering reconstruction of small tubes able to replace a urethra would facilitate largely the work of the urologist surgeons. Indeed they often lack of the necessary tissue for the penile reconstruction surgeries.

Magnan et al.. had demonstrated the feasibility of a human autologous tube (Figure 9) reconstructed on the basis of the well known model of blood vessel engineered by the team of Dr François A. Auger at the LOEX in the 90s [111]. Using self-assembly method, fibroblast sheets were produced in the presence of ascorbic acid and then rolled in a tubular structure (Figure 10). Mechanical characteristics of this model are roughly similar or even better than the ones of the native tissue [107].

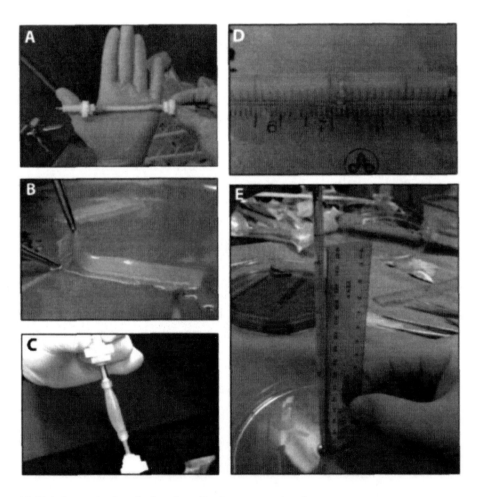

Figure 10. Tubular urethral equivalent from Petri to surgeon hands.
A) Tubular urethral equivalent rolled on a pipette. B) The surgeon can handle the tubular urethral equivalent. C) The tubular urethral equivalent can retain liquid. D) Sutures can be made on this tubular urethral equivalent. E) Sutured tubular structure measuring 14 cm.

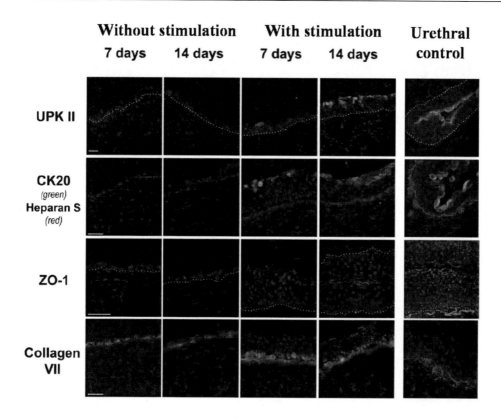

Figure 11. Differentiation of urothelial cells in a tubular urethral equivalent under dynamic conditions (flow). UPKII, CK20, Heparan S, ZO-1 and collagen VII are markers of urothelium maturation. Note the immature differentiation of tubular urethral equivalent in static conditions and the one well differentiated for the dynamic conditions which are roughly similar to the native porcine urethra.

Despite these impressive results, the problem of the adhesion and right differentiation of the urothelium, which is essential to have a functional urethral epithelium, remains. The next step is the work of Cattan et al. [104]. Tubes were placed in constant flow after epithelial cell seeding. Cell culture medium circulated inside the tube and stimulated the differentiation of the urothelial cells. Uroplakins and tight junction proteins were expressed and formed near native structures (Figure 11).

In Rabbits

Before human implantation, the use of animal models is required. In this case, rabbits were chosen due to their roughly similar urethral organisation. With this view and in the same manner of the fibroblasts from pig for the bladder reconstruction, the cell culture conditions must be modified from the one definite for humans. Cells from rabbits have to be cultured according to their own optimal conditions. For example, an increase in the temperatures during culture is required to mimic internal rabbit organism. Some additives salts had to be added, etc...

To produce a tube showing a good rigidity and to compare it with the human model already established by Cattan in 2010 [104] remain the goal of this step. The optimal cell culture conditions for the production of extracellular matrix have been investigated. Several inducers of collagen synthesis, secretion and deposition had been tested with sometimes a little success. Cell seeding technique was also modified with a greater benefit. This extracellular matrix, once produced by the cells themselves, allows strengthening of the constructions.

Because the texture of reconstructed tissues from rabbit cells is different from the one from the human cells, techniques of manipulations for cell or extracellular matrix sheets have to be revised. Apparently, the more the reconstructed tissues are solid and thick, the better they support sutures and surgical manipulations allowing the graft take.

Nevertheless, the production of urethral equivalents reconstructed by tissue engineering in a rabbit model is promising and will doubtless lead research towards the preclinical step, and forward to the human transplantation of the self assembly substitute.

3.4. Vagina

With regards to what has been done so far, it is obvious that some factors are limiting the feasibility of autologous vaginal tissue reimplantation. One of the most important we can see is the necessity of autologous vaginal tissue, which is not always feasible. Also, how could we assume that the biopsied vaginal tissue is tumor-free in a patient aiming toward reconstructive procedure following oncologic exanteration? The cost is surely another limiting-factor considering the technical time needed to produce the tissue. Long-term evolution of the implanted tissue is yet to be known.

Thus, we aim, first, toward production of a completely autologous vaginal tissue by the self-assembly technique, which, to our knowledge, would be the first of its kind in neovaginal tissue engineering. We have to obtain a well-differentiated tissue and prove adequate vaginal histology. Rabbit implantation could possibly be a step toward the surgical approach of reconstructive procedures.

The usage of our vaginal tissue for human immunodeficiency virus (HIV) testing is another avenue and motivation for neovaginal tissue production. A few teams have so far tempted to analyse the permeability or binding of the virus to the mucosa, and others the cellular viability with usage of anti-HIV creams. A lot is still to come in this field of infectious disease prevention research. We think that a viable neovaginal tissue that reproduces the normal human environment brings infinite possibilities in HIV testing and STD prevention.

Conclusion

Tissue engineering is an evolving field of research and these applications, not only to regenerative medicine but also for fundamental investigation, make possible to hope that many issues will find their solutions. Exponential increase in research in genitourinary regenerative medicine has to respond to exponential increase in the number of the pathologies that can be expected with the ageing of the population and development of the obesity and then diabetes in the next decades. The frontier is our imagination. All contributions to the improvement of the life quality of patients are welcome, and all the models depicted in these pages could help. At the moment, self assembly method, because of its unique exogenous material free feature, seems to be the closest to physiological conditions among those available raising the possibility to generate more appropriate tissue for reconstruction and more accurate model for in vitro studies of normal and pathologic mechanisms. We have a dream, the dream of a clinical translation of our research from bench to patients.

References

[1]   Bradley, W.E., G.W. Timm, and F.B. Scott, Innervation of the detrusor muscle and urethra. *Urol Clin North Am,* 1974. *1*(1): p. 3-27.

[2]   Hodson, C.J. and R.S. Cotran, Reflux nephropathy. *Hosp Pract* (Hosp Ed), 1982. *17*(4): p. 133-5, 138-41, 148-56.

[3]   Apodaca, G., The uroepithelium: not just a passive barrier. *Traffic,* 2004. *5*(3): p. 117-28.

[4]   Young, B., et al.., Wheater's Functional Histology: A Text and Colour Atlas, in *Wheater's Functional Histology: A Text and Colour Atlas,* C. Livingstone, Editor. 2006.

[5]   Hynes, R.O., The extracellular matrix: not just pretty *fibrils. Science,* 2009. *326*(5957): p. 1216-9.

[6]   Wilson, C.B., et al.., Extracellular matrix and integrin composition of the normal bladder wall. *World J Urol,* 1996. *14 Suppl 1*: p. S30-7.

[7]   Wiseman, O.J., C.J. Fowler, and D.N. Landon, The role of the human bladder lamina propria myofibroblast. *BJU Int,* 2003. *91*(1): p. 89-93.

[8]   de Groat, W.C. and N. Yoshimura, Afferent nerve regulation of bladder function in health and disease. *Handb Exp Pharmacol,* 2009(194): p. 91-138.

[9]   Kreft, M.E., et al.., Urothelial injuries and the early wound healing response: tight junctions and urothelial cytodifferentiation. *Histochem Cell Biol,* 2005. *123*(4-5): p. 529-39.

[10]   Hudoklin, S., D. Zupancic, and R. Romih, Maturation of the Golgi apparatus in urothelial cells. *Cell Tissue Res,* 2009. *336*(3): p. 453-63.

[11]   Truschel, S.T., et al.., Primary uroepithelial cultures. A model system to analyze umbrella cell barrier function. *J Biol Chem,* 1999. *274*(21): p. 15020-9.

[12]   Veranic, P., R. Romih, and K. Jezernik, What determines differentiation of urothelial umbrella cells? *Eur J Cell Biol,* 2004. *83*(1): p. 27-34.

[13]   Born, M., et al.., The maintenance of the permeability barrier of bladder facet cells requires a continuous fusion of discoid vesicles with the apical plasma membrane. *Eur J Cell Biol,* 2003. *82*(7): p. 343-50.

[14]   Lewis, S.A., Everything you wanted to know about the bladder epithelium but were afraid to ask. *Am J Physiol Renal Physiol,* 2000. *278*(6): p. F867-74.

[15]   Shingai, T., et al.., Implications of nectin-like molecule-2/IGSF4/RA175/SgIGSF/ TSLC1/SynCAM1 in cell-cell adhesion and transmembrane protein localization in epithelial cells. *J Biol Chem,* 2003. *278*(37): p. 35421-7.

[16]   Liang, F.X., et al.., Organization of uroplakin subunits: transmembrane topology, pair formation and plaque composition. *Biochem J,* 2001. *355*(Pt 1): p. 13-8.

[17] Draper, J.W. and R.B. Stark, End results in the replacement of mucous membrane of the urinary bladder with thick-split grafts of skin. *Surgery,* 1956. *39*(3): p. 434-40.

[18] Goldstein, M.B., L.C. Dearden, and V. Gualtieri, Regeneration of subtotally cystectomized bladder patched with omentum: an experimental study in rabbits. *J Urol,* 1967. *97*(4): p. 664-8.

[19] Nguyen, D.H. and M.E. Mitchell, Gastric bladder reconstruction. *Urol Clin North Am,* 1991. *18*(4): p. 649-57.

[20] Andretto, R., et al.., [Experimental cystoplasty in dogs using preserved equine pericardium]. *AMB Rev Assoc Med Bras,* 1981. *27*(5): p. 153-4.

[21] Tariel, E., et al.., [Replacement enterocystoplasty in man (except Hautmann): principles and technical considerations]. *Ann Urol* (Paris), 2006. *40*(6): p. 368-94.

[22] Burbige, K.A. and T.W. Hensle, The complications of urinary tract reconstruction. *J Urol,* 1986. *136*(1 Pt 2): p. 292-7.

[23] Vemulakonda, V.M., et al.., Metastatic adenocarcinoma after augmentation gastrocystoplasty. *J Urol,* 2008. *179*(3): p. 1094-6; discussion 1097.

[24] McDougal, W.S., Metabolic complications of urinary intestinal diversion. J Urol, 1992. *147*(5): p. 1199-208.

[25] Mundy, A.R. and D.E. Nurse, Calcium balance, growth and skeletal mineralisation in patients with cystoplasties. *Br J Urol,* 1992. *69*(3): p. 257-9.

[26] Ali-El-Dein, B., et al.., Late uro-ileal cancer after incorporation of ileum into the urinary tract. *J Urol,* 2002. *167*(1): p. 84-8.

[27] Woodhams, S.D., et al.., Factors causing variation in urinary N-nitrosamine levels in enterocystoplasties. *BJU Int,* 2001. *88*(3): p. 187-91.

[28] Cross, W.R., D.F. Thomas, and J. Southgate, Tissue engineering and stem cell research in urology. *BJU Int,* 2003. *92*(2): p. 165-71.

[29] Hafez, A.T., et al.., Aerosol transfer of bladder urothelial and smooth muscle cells onto demucosalized colonic segments for porcine bladder augmentation in vivo: a 6-week experimental study. *J Urol,* 2005. *174*(4 Pt 2): p. 1663-7; discussion 1667-8.

[30] Perron, J., [Abnormalities of the penis and abnormalities of the end of the urethra: their surgical treatment]. *Soins,* 1969. *14*(8): p. 347-53.

[31] Cecil, A.B., Hypospadias and epispadias; diagnosis and treatment. *Pediatr Clin North Am,* 1955: p. 711-28.

[32] Vyas, P.R., D.R. Roth, and A.D. Perlmutter, Experience with free grafts in urethral reconstruction. *J Urol,* 1987. *137*(3): p. 471-4.

[33] Caldamone, A.A., et al.., Buccal mucosal grafts for urethral reconstruction. *Urology,* 1998. *51*(5A Suppl): p. 15-9.

[34] Rodriguez-Antolin, J., et al.., General tissue characteristics of the lower urethral and vaginal walls in the domestic rabbit. *Int Urogynecol J Pelvic Floor Dysfunct,* 2009. *20*(1): p. 53-60.

[35] Alt, C., et al.., Increased CCL2 expression and macrophage/monocyte migration during microbicide-induced vaginal irritation. *Curr HIV Res,* 2009. *7*(6): p. 639-49.

[36] Bryan, A.L., J.A. Nigro, and V.S. Counseller, One hundred cases of congenital absence of the vagina. *Surg Gynecol Obstet*, 1949. *88*(1): p. 79-86.

[37] Panici, P.B., et al.., Vaginal reconstruction with the Abbe-McIndoe technique: from dermal grafts to autologous in vitro cultured vaginal tissue transplant. *Semin Reprod Med*, 2011. *29*(1): p. 45-54.

[38] Zhao, M., et al.., Use of autologous micromucosa graft for vaginoplasty in vaginal agenesis. *Ann Plast Surg*, 2009. *63*(6): p. 645-9.

[39] Stany, M.P., et al.., The use of acellular dermal allograft for vulvovaginal reconstruction. *Int J Gynecol Cancer*, 2010. *20*(6): p. 1079-81.

[40] Yang, B., et al.., Vaginal reconstruction with sigmoid colon in patients with congenital absence of vagina and menses retention: a report of treatment experience in 22 young women. *Int Urogynecol J*, 2012.

[41] Mure, P.Y., et al.., [Surgical management of congenital adrenal hyperplasia in young girls]. *Prog Urol, 2003. 13*(6): p. 1381-91.

[42] Hendren, W.H. and A. Atala, Use of bowel for vaginal reconstruction. *J Urol*, 1994. *152*(2 Pt 2): p. 752-5; discussion 756-7.

[43] de Souza, J.P., et al.., Vaginal reconstruction with two lower abdominal skin flaps in rabbits: histological and macroscopic evaluation. *Eur J Obstet Gynecol Reprod Biol*, 2012. *160*(2): p. 179-84.

[44] Jeong, S.I., et al.., Morphology of elastic poly(L-lactide-co-epsilon-caprolactone) copolymers and in vitro and in vivo degradation behavior of their scaffolds. *Biomacromolecules, 2004. 5*(4): p. 1303-9.

[45] Jeong, S.I., et al.., In vivo biocompatibilty and degradation behavior of elastic poly(L-lactide-co-epsilon-caprolactone) scaffolds. *Biomaterials*, 2004. *25*(28): p. 5939-46.

[46] Hayami, J.W., et al.., Design and characterization of a biodegradable composite scaffold for ligament tissue engineering. *J Biomed Mater Res A, 2010. 92*(4): p. 1407-20.

[47] Burdick, J.A. and G. Vunjak-Novakovic, Engineered microenvironments for controlled stem cell differentiation. *Tissue Eng Part A,* 2009. *15*(2): p. 205-19.

[48] Salem, A.K., et al.., Interactions of 3T3 fibroblasts and endothelial cells with defined pore features. *J Biomed Mater Res,* 2002. *61*(2): p. 212-7.

[49] Botchwey, E.A., et al.., Tissue engineered bone: measurement of nutrient transport in three-dimensional matrices. *J Biomed Mater Res A,* 2003. *67*(1): p. 357-67.

[50] Rosario, D.J., et al.., Decellularization and sterilization of porcine urinary bladder matrix for tissue engineering in the lower urinary tract. *Regen Med,* 2008. *3*(2): p. 145-56.

[51] Gilbert, T.W., T.L. Sellaro, and S.F. Badylak, Decellularization of tissues and organs. *Biomaterials,* 2006. *27*(19): p. 3675-83.

[52] Sutherland, R.S., et al.., Regeneration of bladder urothelium, smooth muscle, blood vessels and nerves into an acellular tissue matrix. *J Urol,* 1996. *156*(2 Pt 2): p. 571-7.

[53] Reing, J.E., et al.., The effects of processing methods upon mechanical and biologic properties of porcine dermal extracellular matrix scaffolds. *Biomaterials,* 2010. *31*(33): p. 8626-33.

[54] Olde Damink, L.H., et al.., Influence of ethylene oxide gas treatment on the in vitro degradation behavior of dermal sheep collagen. *J Biomed Mater Res,* 1995. *29*(2): p. 149-55.

[55] Brown, B., et al.., The basement membrane component of biologic scaffolds derived from extracellular matrix. *Tissue Eng,* 2006. *12*(3): p. 519-26.

[56] Hodde, J.P., et al.., Vascular endothelial growth factor in porcine-derived extracellular matrix. *Endothelium,* 2001. *8*(1): p. 11-24.

[57] Lantz, G.C., et al.., Small intestinal submucosa as a vascular graft: a review. *J Invest Surg*, 1993. *6*(3): p. 297-310.

[58] Kajbafzadeh, A.M., et al.., Time-dependent neovasculogenesis and regeneration of different bladder wall components in the bladder acellular matrix graft in rats. *J Surg Res*, 2007. *139*(2): p. 189-202.

[59] Oberpenning, F., et al.., De novo reconstitution of a functional mammalian urinary bladder by tissue engineering. *Nat Biotechnol*, 1999. *17*(2): p. 149-55.

[60] Atala, A., et al.., Tissue-engineered autologous bladders for patients needing cystoplasty. *Lancet*, 2006. *367*(9518): p. 1241-6.

[61] Cook, A.D., et al.., *Characterization and development of RGD-peptide*-modified poly(lactic acid-co-lysine) as an interactive, resorbable biomaterial. *J Biomed Mater Res*, 1997. *35*(4): p. 513-23.

[62] Hurst, R.E. and R.B. Bonner, Mapping of the distribution of significant proteins and proteoglycans in small intestinal submucosa by fluorescence microscopy. *J Biomater Sci Polym Ed*, 2001. *12*(11): p. 1267-79.

[63] Ho, K.L., M.N. Witte, and E.T. Bird, 8-ply small intestinal submucosa tension-free sling: spectrum of postoperative inflammation. *J Urol*, 2004. *171*(1): p. 268-71.

[64] Feil, G., et al.., Investigations of urothelial cells seeded on commercially available small intestine submucosa. *Eur Urol*, 2006. *50*(6): p. 1330-7.

[65] Zhang, Y., et al.., Coculture of bladder urothelial and smooth muscle cells on small intestinal submucosa: potential applications for tissue engineering technology. *J Urol*, 2000. *164*(3 Pt 2): p. 928-34; discussion 934-5.

[66] Zhang, Y., et al.., Challenges in a larger bladder replacement with cell-seeded and unseeded small intestinal submucosa grafts in a subtotal cystectomy model. *BJU Int*, 2006. *98*(5): p. 1100-5.

[67] Sievert, K.D. and E.A. Tanagho, Organ-specific acellular matrix for reconstruction of the urinary tract. *World J Urol*, 2000. *18*(1): p. 19-25.

[68] Erdani Kreft, M. and M. Sterle, The effect of lamina propria on the growth and differentiation of urothelial cells in vitro. *Pflugers Arch*, 2000. *440*(5 Suppl): p. R181-2.

[69] Farhat, W.A., et al.., Porcine bladder acellular matrix (ACM): protein expression, mechanical properties. *Biomed Mater*, 2008. *3*(2): p. 025015.

[70] Merguerian, P.A., et al.., Acellular bladder matrix allografts in the regeneration of functional bladders: evaluation of large-segment (> 24 cm) substitution in a porcine model. *BJU Int*, 2000. *85*(7): p. 894-8.

[71] Farhat, W.A. and H. Yeger, Does mechanical stimulation have any role in urinary bladder tissue engineering? *World J Urol*, 2008. *26*(4): p. 301-5.

[72] Olsen, L., et al.., Urethral reconstruction with a new synthetic absorbable device. An experimental study. *Scand J Urol Nephrol*, 1992. *26*(4): p. 323-6.

[73] Italiano, G., et al.., Reconstructive surgery of the urethra: a pilot study in the rabbit on the use of hyaluronan benzyl ester (Hyaff-11) biodegradable grafts. *Urol Res*, 1997. *25*(2): p. 137-42.

[74] Atala, A., et al.., Injectable alginate seeded with chondrocytes as a potential treatment for vesicoureteral reflux. *J Urol*, 1993. *150*(2 Pt 2): p. 745-7.

[75] Atala, A., et al.., Endoscopic treatment of vesicoureteral reflux with a chondrocyte-alginate suspension. *J Urol*, 1994. *152*(2 Pt 2): p. 641-3; discussion 644.

[76]   Diamond, D.A. and A.A. Caldamone, Endoscopic correction of vesicoureteral reflux in children using autologous chondrocytes: preliminary results. *J Urol*, 1999. *162*(3 Pt 2): p. 1185-8.

[77]   Fu, W.J., et al.., Biodegradable urethral stents seeded with autologous urethral epithelial cells in the treatment of post-traumatic urethral stricture: a feasibility study in a rabbit model. *BJU Int*, 2009. *104*(2): p. 263-8.

[78]   Kropp, B.P., et al.., Rabbit urethral regeneration using small intestinal submucosa onlay grafts. *Urology*, 1998. *52*(1): p. 138-42.

[79]   Chen, F., J.J. Yoo, and A. Atala, Acellular collagen matrix as a possible "off the shelf" biomaterial for urethral repair. *Urology*, 1999. *54*(3): p. 407-10.

[80]   De Filippo, R.E., J.J. Yoo, and A. Atala, Urethral replacement using cell seeded tubularized collagen matrices. *J Urol*, 2002. *168*(4 Pt 2): p. 1789-92; discussion 1792-3.

[81]   Dorin, R.P., et al.., Tubularized urethral replacement with unseeded matrices: what is the maximum distance for normal tissue regeneration? *World J Urol*, 2008. *26*(4): p. 323-6.

[82]   Fu, Q., et al.., Urethral replacement using epidermal cell-seeded tubular acellular bladder collagen matrix. *BJU Int*, 2007. *99*(5): p. 1162-5.

[83]   Li, C., et al.., Preliminary experimental study of tissue-engineered urethral reconstruction using oral keratinocytes seeded on BAMG. *Urol Int, 2008. 81*(3): p. 290-5.

[84]   Li, C., et al.., Urethral reconstruction using oral keratinocyte seeded bladder acellular matrix grafts. *J Urol*, 2008. *180*(4): p. 1538-42.

[85]   Parnigotto, P.P., et al.., Experimental defect in rabbit urethra repaired with acellular aortic matrix. *Urol Res*, 2000. *28*(1): p. 46-51.

[86]   Hu, Y.F., et al.., Curative effect and histocompatibility evaluation of reconstruction of traumatic defect of rabbit urethra using extracellular matrix. *Chin J Traumatol*, 2008. *11*(5): p. 274-8.

[87]   Gardner, W.U., Sensitivity of the vagina to estrogen: genetic and transmitted differences. *Ann N Y Acad Sci*, 1959. *83*: p. 145-59.

[88]   Kahn, R.H., Vaginal keratinization in vitro. *Ann N Y Acad Sci*, 1959. *83*: p. 347-55.

[89]   Sobel, J.D., et al.., Human vaginal epithelial multilayer tissue culture. *In Vitro*, 1979. *15*(12): p. 993-1000.

[90]   Iguchi, T., et al.., Growth of normal mouse vaginal epithelial cells in and on collagen gels. *Proc Natl Acad Sci U S A*, 1983. *80*(12): p. 3743-7.

[91]   Iguchi, T., F.D. Uchima, and H.A. Bern, Growth of mouse vaginal epithelial cells in culture: effect of sera and supplemented serum-free media. *In Vitro Cell Dev Biol*, 1987. *23*(8): p. 535-40.

[92]   Uchima, F.D., et al.., Estrogen and progestin receptors in mouse vaginal epithelium and fibromuscular wall. *Biochim Biophys Acta*, 1985. *841*(1): p. 135-8.

[93]   Yang, J., et al.., Sustained growth in primary culture of normal mammary epithelial cells embedded in collagen gels. *Proc Natl Acad Sci U S A*, 1980. *77*(4): p. 2088-92.

[94]   Uchima, F.D., et al.., Growth of mouse vaginal epithelial cells in culture: functional integrity of the estrogen receptor system and failure of estrogen to induce proliferation. *Cancer Lett*, 1987. *35*(3): p. 227-35.

[95]   Turyk, M.E., et al.., Growth and characterization of epithelial cells from normal human uterine ectocervix and endocervix. *In Vitro Cell Dev Biol*, 1989. *25*(6): p. 544-56.

[96] Doillon, C.J., A. Altchek, and F.H. Silver, Method of growing vaginal mucosal cells on a collagen sponge matrix. Results of preliminary studies. *J Reprod Med,* 1990. *35*(3): p. 203-7.

[97] Zong, W., et al.., Regulation of MMP-1 by sex steroid hormones in fibroblasts derived from the female pelvic floor. *Am J Obstet Gynecol,* 2007. *196*(4): p. 349 e1-11.

[98] Zong, W., L.A. Meyn, and P.A. Moalli, The amount and activity of active matrix metalloproteinase 13 is suppressed by estradiol and progesterone in human pelvic floor fibroblasts. *Biol Reprod,* 2009. *80*(2): p. 367-74.

[99] Panici, P.B., et al.., Vaginoplasty using autologous in vitro cultured vaginal tissue in a patient with Mayer-von-Rokitansky-Kuster-Hauser syndrome. *Hum Reprod,* 2007. *22*(7): p. 2025-8.

[100] Hjelm, B.E., et al.., Development and characterization of a three-dimensional organotypic human vaginal epithelial cell model. *Biol Reprod,* 2010. *82*(3): p. 617-27.

[101] Dorin, R.P., A. Atala, and R.E. Defilippo, Bioengineering a vaginal replacement using a small biopsy of autologous tissue. *Semin Reprod Med,* 2011. *29*(1): p. 38-44.

[102] Bouhout, S., et al.., In vitro reconstruction of an autologous, watertight, and resistant vesical equivalent. *Tissue Eng Part* A, 2010. *16*(5): p. 1539-48.

[103] Bouhout, S., et al.., Bladder substitute reconstructed in a physiological pressure environment. *J Pediatr Urol,* 2011. *7*(3): p. 276-82.

[104] Cattan, V., et al.., Mechanical stimuli-induced urothelial differentiation in a human tissue-engineered tubular genitourinary graft. *Eur Urol,* 2011. *60*(6): p. 1291-8.

[105] Imbeault, A., et al.., Surgical option for the correction of Peyronie's disease: an autologous tissue-engineered endothelialized graft. *J Sex Med,* 2011. *8*(11): p. 3227-35.

[106] Magnan, M., et al.., In vitro reconstruction of a tissue-engineered endothelialized bladder from a single porcine biopsy. *J Pediatr Urol,* 2006. *2*(4): p. 261-70.

[107] Magnan, M., et al.., Tissue engineering of a genitourinary tubular tissue graft resistant to suturing and high internal pressures. *Tissue Eng Part A,* 2009. *15*(1): p. 197-202.

[108] Ouellet, G., et al.., Production of an optimized tissue-engineered pig connective tissue for the reconstruction of the urinary tract. *Tissue Eng Part A,* 2011. *17*(11-12): p. 1625-33.

[109] Auger, F.A., et al.., A truly new approach for tissue engineering: the LOEX self-assembly technique. *Ernst Schering Res Found Workshop,* 2002(35): p. 73-88.

[110] Auger, F.A., et al.., Tissue-engineered skin substitutes: from in vitro constructs to in vivo applications. *Biotechnol Appl Biochem,* 2004. *39*(Pt 3): p. 263-75.

[111] L'Heureux, N., et al.., A human tissue-engineered vascular media: a new model for pharmacological studies of contractile responses. *Faseb J,* 2001. *15*(2): p. 515-24.

[112] Carrier, P., et al.., Impact of cell source on human cornea reconstructed by tissue engineering. *Invest Ophthalmol Vis Sci,* 2009. *50*(6): p. 2645-52.

[113] Trottier, V., et al.., IFATS collection: Using human adipose-derived stem/stromal cells for the production of new skin substitutes. *Stem Cells,* 2008. *26*(10): p. 2713-23.

[114] Vermette, M., et al.., Production of a new tissue-engineered adipose substitute from human adipose-derived stromal cells. *Biomaterials,* 2007. *28*(18): p. 2850-60.

[115] Corriveau, M.P., et al.., The fibrotic phenotype of systemic sclerosis fibroblasts varies with disease duration and severity of skin involvement: reconstitution of skin fibrosis development using a tissue engineering approach. *J Pathol,* 2009. *217*(4): p. 534-42.

[116] Jean, J., et al.., Development of an in vitro psoriatic skin model by tissue engineering. J *Dermatol Sci,* 2009. *53*(1): p. 19-25.

[117] Simon, F., et al.., *Enhanced secretion of TIMP-1 by human hypertrophic scar keratinocytes could contribute to fibrosis.* Burns, 2011.

[118] Germain, L., et al.., Improvement of human keratinocyte isolation and culture using thermolysin. *Burns,* 1993. *19*(2): p. 99-104.

[119] Kreft, M.E., et al.., Formation and maintenance of blood-urine barrier in urothelium. *Protoplasma,* 2010. *246*(1-4): p. 3-14.

[120] Yoshimura, K., et al.., Characterization of freshly isolated and cultured cells derived from the fatty and fluid portions of liposuction aspirates. *J Cell Physiol,* 2006. *208*(1): p. 64-76.

[121] Ebrahimian, T.G., et al.., Plasminogen activator inhibitor-1 controls bone marrow-derived cells therapeutic effect through MMP9 signaling: role in physiological and pathological wound healing. *Stem Cells,* 2012. *30*(7): p. 1436-46.

[122] Salcedo, R., et al.., Vascular endothelial growth factor and basic fibroblast growth factor induce expression of CXCR4 on human endothelial cells: In vivo neovascularization induced by stromal-derived factor-1alpha. *Am J Pathol,* 1999. *154*(4): p. 1125-35.

[123] Ebrahimian, T.G., et al.., *Cell therapy based on adipose tissue-derived stromal cells promotes physiological and pathological wound healing. Arterioscler Thromb Vasc Biol,* 2009. *29*(4): p. 503-10.

[124] Blasi, A., et al.., Dermal fibroblasts display similar phenotypic and differentiation capacity to fat-derived mesenchymal stem cells, but differ in anti-inflammatory and angiogenic potential. *Vasc Cell,* 2011. *3*(1): p. 5.

[125] Park, H.K., et al.., Adipose-derived stromal cells inhibit allergic airway inflammation in mice. *Stem Cells Dev,* 2010. *19*(11): p. 1811-8.

In: Handbook of Genitourinary Medicine: New Research   ISBN: 978-1-62618-226-4
Editor: Rashmi R. Singh   © 2013 Nova Science Publishers, Inc.

Chapter VII

Chemotherapy in Invasive Bladder Cancer

Nabil Ismaili[*]

Department of Oncology and Radiotherapy, Medical Oncology, Oncology Center,
University Hospital Mohammed VI, and Faculty of Medicine,
Cadi Ayyad University, Marrakech, Morocco

Abstract

A systematic study has been undertaken of the role of chemotherapy in the treatment of invasive bladder cancer (localized and metastatic). Bladder cancer is the seventh most common cancer and the ninth most common cause of cancer deaths for men worldwide. Transitional cell carcinoma is the most predominant histological type. Cystectomy with pelvic lymph nodes dissection is the standard local treatment of muscle invasive bladder cancer (T2–T4); the anatomical extent of pelvic lymphadenectomy is not accurately defined. Bladder cancer is highly chemosensitive. In the last decade, chemotherapy was introduced as part of the management of the disease. Randomized trials and metaanalyses confirmed the survival benefit of neoadjuvant chemotherapy before local treatment, consequently, this sequence should be considered as standard treatment of choice, for patients with good performance status (0–1) and good renal function–glomerular filtration rate (GFR) [60 mL/min]. The benefit of adjuvant chemotherapy is not clear. For patients treated with primary surgery, adjuvant chemotherapy is a valuable option in the case of lymph nodes involvement. In metastatic setting, chemotherapy based on cisplatin should be considered as standard treatment of choice for patients with good performance status (0-1) and good renal function-glomerular filtration rate (GFR) > 60 mL/min. The standard treatment is based on cisplatin chemotherapy regimens type MVAC, HD-MVAC, gemcitabine plus cisplatin (GC) or dose dense GC. In unfit patients, carboplatin based regimes; gemcitabine plus carboplatin or methotrexate plus carboplatin plus vinblastine (MCAVI) are reasonable options. Vinflunine and gemcitabine-paclitaxel are two reasonable therapeutic options in patients with cisplatin refractory disease. Future

---

[*] E-mail address: ismailinabil@yahoo.fr

prospects for the targeted therapies in the management of invasive bladder cancer will be discussed.

I. Introduction

It is the intent of this paper to summarize what is known about the role of chemotherapy in the management of bladder cancer (neoadjuvant, adjuvant and palliative chemotherapy). The role of targeted therapies in metastatic bladder transitional cell carcinoma will be reviewed. Systemic treatment of other histological types such as squamous cell carcinoma, adenocarcinoma, *lymphoma, sarcoma and small cell carcinoma are not discussed in this chapter*. The incidence of bladder cancer is increasing. An estimated 386,300 new cases and 150,200 deaths from bladder cancer occurred in 2008 worldwide [1]. The highest incidence is observed in Egypt with 37 cases per 100,000 inhabitants [2]. Bladder cancer occurs in the majority of cases in males with a male/female sex ratio of 3:1. It represents the seventh most common cancer for men [1]. In Morocco, bladder cancer was the sixth most common cancer in 2005 according to Rabat registry. The average age of diagnosis is 65 years [3]. Smoking is the most implicated risk factor in western countries, followed by other factors such as polycyclic aromatic hydrocarbons and cyclophosphamide [2]. In East Africa (especially Egypt), chronic infection with *Schistosoma haematobium* is the most common etiology and is often associated with squamous cell carcinoma [1,2]. Transitional cell carcinoma (TCC) is the most predominant histological type which represents more than 90% of the cases [4]. In more than 70% of the cases, the diagnosis is made at early stage of the disease (stages Ta and T1). Bladder tumors are called muscle invasive (cT2) when they infiltrate the bladder muscle. The standard treatment in this setting is radical cystectomy with pelvic lymphadenectomy; the anatomical extent of pelvic lymphadenectomy has not accurately been defined so far (NCCN 2011). However, half of the patients develop distant metastasis and die of the disease. In the last decade, the management of these tumors had become multidisciplinary, often involving perioperative chemotherapy (neoadjuvant or adjuvant). Fifty percent of the patients with the disease at advanced stages (T2 or more) experience metastatic relapse. In metastatic setting, chemotherapy treatment remains the only therapeutic option. It has the objective to alleviate the symptoms, to improve quality of life and to improve survival. In bladder TCC, chemotherapy showed very little progress and the standard MVAC is still the most used regimen and that since several years.

II. Literature Review

The literature review was conducted by using PUBMED data base using the following keywords: bladder cancer, transitional cell carcinoma, chemotherapy, cisplatin, and targeted therapies. The abstracts of papers presented at the annual meeting of the American Society of Medical Oncology (ASCO) were also analyzed. All Phase III trials were considered. The most important phase II trials have been also included in our article. The research was carried out from January 1980 until December 2011.

III. Prognostic Factors in Metastatic Setting

A. In First Line

Performance status (≤70%) and liver metastases are recognized as independent factors of poor prognosis in first line metastatic setting. In a retrospective review of 203 patients managed with chemotherapy, the median survival was 33, 13.4 and 9.3 months respectively, in patients with 0, 1, and 2 factors, respectively ($p = 0,0001$) [5]. Prognostic factors helps better to define the therapeutic strategy. For patients with two factors, it is suggested that aggressive chemotherapy should be avoided because of an increased risk of toxicity [5].

B. In Second Line

Performance status (> 0), hemoglobin level (< 10 g/L), and liver metastasis are recognized as independent factors of poor prognosis in second line metastatic setting according to a recent prospective study. The median overall survival (OS) of 370 patients treated with chemotherapy for TCC carcinoma of the bladder with 0, 1, 2 and 3 factors were 14.2, 7.3, 3.8, and 1.7 months ($P < 0.001$), respectively [6].

IV. Chemotherapy in Metastatic Disease

A. Single Agents

Bladder TCC are chemosensitive tumors. However, the response to a single agent is limited. Cisplatin is one of the most active drugs that give the highest overall response rate (ORR). Other drugs are also active (Table 1).

Table 1. ORR of single agents

Drugs	ORR
Cisplatin	33%
Methotrexate	29%
Doxorubicin	23%
5-fluoro-uracil	35%
Vinblastine	-
Cyclophosphamide	-
Mitomycine C	21%
Carboplatin	12-14%
Gemcitabine	24-28%
Paclitaxel	10-40%
Docetaxel	13-31%
Vinflunine	15%
Eribulin	38%
ORR : Overall response rate	

B. Multi-agents Chemotherapy

1. Cisplatin-based Chemotherapy

a. Conventional Regimens

The first protocols based on cisplatin (CMV: cisplatin, cyclophosphamide and vinblastine; and CISCA: cisplatin, doxorubicin and cyclophosphamide) resulted in 12 to 78% ORR. The two protocols CMV and CISCA were widely used in the 1980s but did not show superiority in survival versus cisplatin alone [7-10]. Since 1990, the MVAC has been considered as a standard first-line therapy in metastatic disease. This regimen was for the first time studied in a nonrandomized phase II trial by Sternberg and colleagues in 1985 [11,12] and concerned 25 patients. They showed a sustained ORR in 71% of the cases and 50% of complete responses (CR). Two randomized phase III trials demonstrated the superiority of the MVAC to CISCA and CDDP, respectively, both in ORR, and in OS [13,14]. The MVAC is efficient, but particularly toxic. In the phase II study [11], the combination induced one toxic death and 4 febrile neutropenias (16%), in addition to vomiting, anorexia, mucositis (grade 3-4 in 22% of the cases), alopecia and renal insufficiency. To improve the results obtained with the MVAC, an intensification of this same protocol as HD-MVAC was tested in a phase III EORTC trial including more than 250 patients. In the experimental arm, all drugs were administered in day 1 and day 14. Prevention of toxicity was based on the routine use of Granulocyte Colony-Stimulating Factors (GCS-F). Although the OS which represents the primary end point of the study, was identical in the two arms at 7.3 years median follow-up. However, the study showed that the intensification of the protocol improved CR (25 vs. 10%) and progression-free survival (PFS) (9.5 vs. 8.1 months, p = 0.03). Survivals at 2 and 5 years were also better (37% -22% vs. 25-22%, respectively). In addition, the systematic use of GCSF made the HD-MVAC better tolerated. While the primary end point was not achieved, the intensified MVAC is widely used in metastatic settings [15,16]. Table 2 summarizes the results of the most important phase III trials investigating first line chemotherapy in advanced bladder TCC.

b. Second Generation Drugs

*Gemcitabine Based Regimens
In the 1990s, gemcitabine was a new molecule in the treatment of bladder TCC.

The first phase II trials evaluating the use of gemcitabine as single agent showed an improvement of ORR by 24 to 28%. The combination of gemcitabine with cisplatin (GC) has further improved these results with higher ORR (57%) and CR (15 to 21%) [17]. Based on these encouraging results, a phase III trial was conducted to compare the GC protocol to the standard MVAC. The study was designed to demonstrate superiority of the experimental arm in OS. The results showed no improvement of OS (MVAC: 14.8 months vs. GC: 13.8 months) and ORR (MVAC: 45.7 vs. GC: 49.4%). But due to the better safety profile, the GC was considered not inferior to MVAC [18,19]. A recent phase III trial compared the intensified HD-MVAC (n = 118) to the dose dense GC (DD-GC) (n = 57) (G: 2500 mg/m^2, C: 70 mg/m^2 q 2 wks). The results were presented at the ASCO 2011 and showed that efficacy was similar in both treatments (ORR = 47.4 vs. 47.4%, respectively: p = 0.9; and OS

= 18.4 vs. 20.7 months, respectively: p = 0.7), however, the safety profile was slightly better in favor to DD-GC [20].

Table 2. Phase III trials investigating first line chemotherapy treatments in metastatic bladder cancer

Authors	Years	Phase	Treatment	No	Results	Toxicity
Logothetis [13]	1990	III	MVAC vs CISCA	120	Sup	Sup
Loehrer [14]	1992	III	MVAC vs Cisplatin	146	Sup	Sup
Von der Maase [18,19]	2000	III	MVAC vs GC	405	Equivalents	Sup
Sternberg [15,16]	2001	III	MVAC-HD vs MVAC	259	Equivalents	Inf
Bamias [26]	2004	III	MVAC vs DC	120	Sup	-
Dreicer [31]	2004	III	MVAC vs PCa	85	Interupted early	Sup
Bellmunt [48]	2007	III	PCG vs GC	627	Equivalents	Sup
De Santis [37]	2010	III	GCa vs MCAVI	238	Equivalents	Inf
Bamias [20]	2011	III	DD-GC vs MVAC-HD	175	Equivalents	Inf

Abbreviations. JCO : Journal of Clinical Oncology; MVAC : methotrexat-vinblastine-doxorubicin-cisplatin; CISCA: cisplatin-cyclophosphamide-doxorubicin; DC: docetaxel plus cisplatin; PCG : paclitaxel-cisplatin-gemcitabin; PCa : paclitaxel plus carboplatin; MCAVI : methotrexate-carboplatin-vinblastine; HD : high dose; DD : dose dance; ORR : objective response rate; OS : overall survival; PFS : progression free survival.

*Taxanes Based Regimens

Cisplatin was also tested in phase II studies with other new drugs, particularly with taxanes (Table 3). The combination of cisplatin with paclitaxel and cisplatin with docetaxel improved ORR by 50-70% and 52-62%, respectively [21-25]. We note that these combinations remain inferior to the standard chemotherapy as was proven by the phase III randomized study conducted by the Hellenic Cooperative Oncology Group comparing docetaxel-cisplatin to MVAC. The standard protocol was superior in ORR (54.2% vs. 37.4%, p = 0.017), time to progression (TTP) (9.4 vs. 6.1 months, p = 0.003) and OS (14.2 vs. 9.3 months, p = 0.026) [26].

Table 3. Taxane based regimens (phase 2 trials)

Auteur	Protocols	N	Results		
			ORR (%)	TTP (months)	OS (months)
Burch [21]	PC	34	70%	-	-
Dreicer [22]	PC	52	50	-	10.6
Dimopoulos [23]	DC	66	52%	5	8
DelMuro et al. [24]	DC	38	58	6.9	10.4
Sengelov et al. [25]	DC	25	60	-	13.6

PC : paclitaxel-cisplatin; DC : docetaxel-cisplatin; ORR : overall response rate; OS : overall survival; TTP : time to progression.

2. Chemotherapy Doublets Based on other Platinum Drugs

Carboplatin is not as efficient as cisplatin. But has the advantage of being easily administered and better tolerated. Therefore, carboplatin-based protocols should be considered in patient ineligible (unfit) for cisplatin-based chemotherapy (Table 4) [27]. Carboplatin has been tested with paclitaxel in several phase II trials and permitted to achieve more than 63% ORR, but CR was limited as compared to cisplatin based protocols. Based on these frustrating results and other data suggesting the limited activity of this protocol [29,30], a phase III study was stopped early due to lack of recruitment. This study was designed to compare paclitaxel-carboplatin to MVAC [31]. Gemcitabine used in combination with carboplatin showed significantly lower results than cisplatin plus gemcitabine. ORR was high (59%), but the comparison with the GC showed that the standard arm was significantly better according to the results of one randomized phase II study [32-35]. Oxaliplatin is another platinum drug which showed only marginal activity as monotherapy [36]. In another hand, the EORTC conducted a phase III trial comparing unfit patients having metastatic TCC, the protocol based on carboplatin (AUC 4.5 on day) - gemcitabine (1000 mg/m^2 on day 1 and day 8) (GCa), repeated every 21 days, to the protocol M-CAVI [methotrexate (30 mg/m^2 on day 1, day 15, and day 22), carboplatin (AUC 4.5 on day 1) and vinblastine (3 mg/m^2 on day 1, day 15, and day 22)], repeated every 28 days. The results presented at ASCO 2010, confirmed the equivalence in OS between the 2 treatments, with a better toxicity profile in favor to the GCa protocol [37].

Table 4. Carboplatin based doublets (phase 2 trials)

Author	Protocol	No	Results		
			ORR	TTP	OS (months)
Redman [28]	PCa	35	51%	-	9.5
Small [29]	PCa	29	20.7	4	9
Vaughn [30]	PCa	33	50%	-	-
Bellmun [32]	GCa	16	44%	-	-
Nogue-Aliguer [33]	GCa	41	56.1	7.2	10.1
Shannon [34]	GCa	17	58.8	4.6	10.5
Dogliotti [35]	GCa vs GC (Randomized phase II)	110	CR : 1.8% vs 14.5%	-	9.8 vs 12.8

Abbreviations. PCa : paclitaxel-carboplatin; GCa : gemcitabine-carboplatin; GC : gemcitabine-cisplatin; RO : objective response rate; OS : overall survivall; PFS: progression free survivall.

3. Doublets without Platinum Drugs

Data on the effectiveness of drugs, in patients with good or poor condition are not sufficient. The literature reports only phase II trials with low number of patients. The protocol which is most studied is based on gemcitabine in combination with other molecules. Gemcitabine-paclitaxel combination appears to produce a significant improvement. This protocol improved ORR to 40-60% [38-40]. Several schemes were tested. A phase II study investigated the gemcitabine-paclitaxel weekly, showed an ORR of up to 69% (42% of CR), however the rate of grade 3-4 pulmonary toxicity and toxic death is high. Therefore, the authors recommended disregard the use of this regimen in practice [41]. With docetaxel, gemcitabine is active and well tolerated. In 3 different phase II studies the ORR was between

30 and 50% [42-44]. Gemcitabine was also evaluated in association with pemetrexed in 2 phases II trials in 64 and 44 patients, respectively. The ORR was 20 and 28%. But this combination was very hematotoxic. In addition, 2 toxic deaths were reported [45,46].

Tableau 5. Triplets and sequential regimens (phases II trials)

Author	Protocol	N (phase)	Results			
			CR (%)	PR (%)	TTP (months)	OS (months)
Bellmunt [47]	CPG	58 (phase 1)	27.6	50	-	24
Bajorin [49]	ITP	44	23	45	-	20
Hussain [50]	CaPG	49	32	36	-	14.7
Hainsworth [51]	CaPG	60	12	31	-	11
Edelman [52]	M-CaP (GCSF)	33	0	40	-	-
Tu [53]	M-CP	25 (second line)	56%		-	15.5
Law [54]	M-GP	20	30	15	6.3	18
Pectasides [55]	EDC	30	30	36.7	-	14.5
Dodd [56]	AG → ITP (with GCSF)	14	21	42	-	-
Novick [57]	AG → ITCa (with GCSF)	21	5	19	-	-

ITP: ifosfamide-paclitaxel-cisplatin; CPG : Cisplatin-Paclitaxel-Gemcitabine; CaPG : Carboplatin-Paclitaxel-Gemcitabine; M-CaP : Methotrexate-Carboplatin-Paclitaxel; M-CP : Methotexate-Cisplatin-Paclitaxel; M-GP : Methotrexate Gemcitabine-Paclitaxel; EDC : Epirubicine-Docetaxel-Cisplatine; AG : doxorubicine-cisplatin; ITCa : ifosfamide-paclitaxel-carboplatin; CR : complate response; PR : partial response; ORR : objective response rate; OS : overall survival; PFS : progression free survival.

4. Triplets

To improve the ORR, several phase II and III studies were conducted by testing the addition of a third drug to the standard protocols used in practice. Paclitaxel, in combination with GC, was the first triplet studied in a phase II trial conducted by Bellmunt, showing 77.6% ORR in 58 patients (ORR = 27.6% and PR = 50%) [47]. Therefore, the authors concluded the feasibility and the activity of this triple association. This was the background of a phase III randomized trial developed by the EORTC group, comparing the same protocol to the standard protocol GC. The authors considered the OS as a primary endpoint. Even with significant superiority in ORR for the experimental arm (57.1 vs. 46.4%, p = 0.02), the primary objective of the study was not achieved (OS = 15.7 vs. 12.8 months, p = 0.12, PFS = 8.4 vs. 7.7 months, p = 0.01) [48]. Bajorin has evaluated the feasibility and safety of paclitaxel, ifosfamide and cisplatin triplet administered every 3 weeks in a phase II study. Among 44 evaluable patients, the rate of CR was 23% and PR was 45%. The median survival was 20 months [49]. Paclitaxel-carboplatin-gemcitabine triplet was investigated in two phase II trials involving patients in the first line in one trial, and in 1st/2nd lines in another trial. ORRs and CR were equal to 43-68%, and 32-12%, respectively. The OS was equal to 14.7 and 11 months, respectively [50,51]. Other combinations including paclitaxel have also been reported in the literature, and showed promising activity and acceptable toxicity profile, but, more investigations are required in clinical trials [52-54]. The cisplatin-epirubicin-docetaxel triplet gave 30% complete responses in first line in 30 evaluable patients. The ORR was 66.7%. The median survival reached 14.5 months. The overall safety profile was comparable to MVAC [55].

5. Sequential Protocols

Based on the effectiveness of the sequential regimens in breast cancer, this option was studied in metastatic bladder cancer. In a phase II trial, the doublet doxorubicin-gemcitabine was evaluated in sequence with the triplet paclitaxel-ifosfamide-cisplatin in previously untreated patients (n = 60) with advanced TCC, with the systematic use of GCSF. In the final results recently published, the authors conclude that the regimen is active; however, it is associated with high rate of grade 3-4 hematological toxicity and does not clearly offer a benefit compared with the standard treatments [56]. In another trial, 25 patients with advanced urothelial carcinoma who were ineligible for cisplatin, received doses-dense sequential treatment with doxorubicin plus gemcitabine followed by paclitaxel plus carboplatin. ORR was 56% and the treatment was well tolerated [57]. Table 5 summarizes the most important prospective studies evaluating the role of triplet and sequential regimens.

C. Second and Third Line Chemotherapy

After failure of cisplatin-based first-line therapy, there was no consensus in the management of cisplatin resistant disease. Taxanes (paclitaxel and docetaxel), vinflunine, and antifolate compounds (trimetrexate, piritrexim, and pemetrexed) resulted in 7 to 23% ORR. The FOLFOX4 was also studied in a phase II trial and resulted in 19% ORR [58-60]. In a recent published case study, the authors obtained a CR with FOLFOX4 chemotherapy in a metastatic urothelial cancer patient, after failure of GC combination [61]. The first phase III trial on cisplatin refractory setting compared vinflunine to best supportive care. Vinflunine is a semi-synthetic, vinca-alkaloid compound that targets the microtubules. It was used at a dose of 320 mg/m^2 repeated every 21 days until progression or intolerance. Compared with the control arm, vinflunine was superior in OS > 2 months, however significant grade 3-4 hematologic toxicities (6% of febrile neutropenia, one toxic death, anemia, and thrombocytopenia) were noted [62]. The second phase III trial was designed to compare a short-term (six cycles: arm A) versus prolonged (until progression: arm B) second-line combination chemotherapy of gepcitabine-paclitaxel. On prolonged treatment, more patients experienced severe anemia (arm A: 6.7% versus arm B: 26.7% grade 3-4 anemia; P = 0.011). Therefore, the authors concluded that it was not feasible to deliver a prolonged regimen. However, a high response rate of 40% makes the short protocol (6 cycles) a promising second line treatment option for patients with metastatic TCC [63].

D. New Molecule

Eribulin is a new agent targeting the microtubules, being tested in several primary tumors. In advanced or metastatic TCC, this molecule was evaluated in a phase II trial, and showed a very interesting antitumor activity in front line with 38% ORR. The PFS was estimated to 3.9 months and the safety profile was acceptable (neutropenia, neuropathy, hypoglycemia, and hyponatremia) [64]. Based on these results, a phase III trial is undergoing to compare the standard GC to the combination of GC to Eribulin.

Table 6. Selected phase II trials evaluating the role of targeted therapies

Organization	Treatment	No	Results				Most common grades 3-4 toxicities
			CR (%)	PR (%)	TTP (mo)	OS (mo)	
Hoosier Oncology Group [65]	GC + Bevacizumab	43	21	51	8.2	20.4	Hematological, thromboembolism
USA (Texas) [69]	GC + sunutinib	15	Interrupted for adverse events				Hematological++
Espagne [70]	Sunitinib	37	8%		5.6	-	Fatigue, HT, H-F syndrome
Allemagne [72]	GC ± sorafenib	85	82 vs 78		6.3 vs 7.2	-	Hematological
NCI Trial [78]	Trastuzumab + CaPG	44 (HER2+++)	11	59		14	Haematological, sensory neuropathy, cardiac
CALGB [80]	Gefitinib + GC	58	48		7	15	Hematological, skin rash, diarrhea,
Allemagne [81]	Lapatinib	59 (second line)	0	3	8.6 weeks	-	Diarrhea, vomiting, dehydration
Italy and USA [82]	Everolimus	45 (second line)	0	8	3.3	10.5	Hematological, fatigue, metabolic, mucositis

GC : Gemcitabine-Cisplatin; ORR : objective response rate; RC : complete response; PR : partial response; S : stabilisation; DR : disease control; PFS : progression free survival; OS : overall survival; CaPG : Paclitaxel-Gemcitabine-Carboplatin.

E. Targeted Therapies

Despite the promising results obtained by chemotherapy based on MVAC or GC, the majority of patients die of metastatic disease. The new progress in molecular biology has prompted the investigators to evaluate several molecules in metastatic bladder TCC. Overexpression of several receptors such as the VEGFR (vascular endothelial growth factor receptor) on endothelial cells, the EGFR (epidermal growth factor receptor, the PDGFR (platlet derived growth factor receptor), and the FGFR (fibroblast growth factor receptor), on tumor cells, led the investigators to evaluate the efficacy and safety of new molecules targeting signaling pathways controlled by these proteins in metastatic setting. Deregulated signaling pathways and targeted therapy in bladder cancer. The role of targeted therapy alone, in combination with chemotherapy, and in maintenance was evaluated using different molecules (bevacizumab, sunitinib, sorafenib, pazopanib, dovitinib, vandetanib, trastuzumab, cetuximab, erlotinib, lapatinib, everolimus, bortezomibe) (Table 6) [65-84].

1. Targeting Angiogenesis

Increased signaling through VEGFR and FGFR characterizes many TCC tumors and increased tumor vascularization. Angiogenesis is a very important step to tumor growth, invasion and metastasis. Therefore, targeting angiogenesis is a very interesting strategy which can be achieved by the use of monoclonal antibodies or by using small molecules tyrosine kinase inhibitors.

a. Monoclonal Antibodies

*Bevacizumab

Bevacizumab is a humanized monoclonal antibody (mAb) targeting the VEGF (Vascular Endothelial Factor) which has been approved by FDA in combination with chemotherapy as a standard treatment in first line and second line in different metastatic tumors. In bladder TCC, bevacizumab (15 mg/kg on day 1) was evaluated in first line treatment in combination with GC protocol (gemcitabine 1250 on D1 and D8 and cisplatin 70 mg/m^2 on D1, the cycle was repeated every 21 days) in a phase II trial (45 patients). Mature data presented at ASCO 2010 showed similar results in ORR and PFS to those obtained by the GC protocol, but OS was superior estimated to 20.4 months. A phase III trial comparing GC to GC plus bevacizumab is undergoing [66].

b. Small Molecules

*SU11248 Sunitinib Sutent [®]

Sunitinib is a small molecule playing as a multi-target intracellular tyrosine kinases inhibitor by inhibiting multiple receptors (EGFR, VERFR-1/2, C-KIT, PDGFR α/β) and the FLT3 and RET kinases. This drug has been approved by the FDA in the front line treatment of metastatic renal cell carcinoma and in the second line treatment of GIST (gastrointestinal stromal tumors) after failure of imatinib. Sunitinib has been tested in bladder cancer as single agent, in combination with chemotherapy, and in maintenance, and showed an interesting anti-tumor activity [67-71]. In a phase II trial presented at ASCO 2010, the Sunitinib was evaluated in association with the GC, but the trial was stopped because of high rate of hematological toxicity [70]. In another phase II study also presented at ASCO 2010, including 33 unfit patients treated with single agent sunitinib, the TTP was estimated to 4.8 months and the clinical benefit to 67%, confirming the role of the angiogenic pathway as an interesting target in the treatment of bladder TCC [71].

*BAY43-9006 Sorafenib Nexavar [®]

Sorafenib is another small multi-target molecule (B-Raf, c-Raf, VEGFR-2/3, VEGFR-3, PDGFR-β) which has been approved by the FDA in second line treatment of metastatic renal cell carcinoma after failure of immunotherapy, and in first line treatment of advanced hepatocellular carcinoma, Child A. It has been tested in bladder TCC as single agent and in combination with chemotherapy in first and second line metastatic disease. However,

Sorafenib didn't have activity in monotherapy [72], and in the combination with GC. Sorafenib did not improve the results of the standard GC in a recent randomized phase II trial [73].

*TKI258 Dovitinib

Dovitinib is an oral drug that inhibits angiogenic factors, including the FGFR and the VEGFR. TKI258, administered at a dose of 500 mg/day taken 5 days per week dosing schedule, was evaluated in phase II trial in second line treatment. The results of this trial, presented this year at the ASCO 2011, are promising [74].

2. EGFR Inhibitors

a. Monoclonal Antibodies

* Trastuzumab

The amplification of the HER2/neu oncogene has been correlated in bladder cancer to a more aggressive disease [75]. Bladder tumors with HER2 amplification represent 10-50% of cases [76-78]. In a multicenter U.S. Phase II study, trastuzumab was tested in combination with paclitaxel-carboplatin-gemcitabine triplet. The study included 109 patients, 57 (52%) had HER2 amplification, and 54 of 57 patients were treated with trastuzumab. The main toxicities were hematological, neurological and cardiac. ORR rate was equal to 70%. The TTP was 9.3 months and OS was14.1 months [79].

b. Small Molecules

*Gefetinib ZD1839 IRESSA ®

Gefitinib is a small molecule tyrosine kinase inhibitor that has been approved by the FDA in the front line treatment of metastatic non small cell lung cancer with activated EGFR mutation. In bladder cancer, it was in the first time evaluated as monotherapy in second-line therapy. This study showed no ORR. Median PFS was limited [80]. Gefitinib was also studied with GC in first line treatment of TCC. However, the results were similar to the GC and MVAC (CALGB 90102) [81].

*GW 572016 Lapatinib Tykerb ®

Lapatinib is a small molecule tyrosine kinase inhinitor allowing the inhibition of HER1 and HER2 receptors. This molecule has been approved by the FDA in the treatment of HER2-positive metastatic breast cancer. In one study, 59 patients with HER2 and/or EGFR amplifications were treated after failure of one or more therapeutic lines. In this phase 2 trial, only one patient (3%) had a partial response and 4 (12%) had stable disease [82].

3. mTOR Inhibitors

The mammalian target of rapamycin (mTOR) is an intracellular serine/threonine protein kinase positioned at a central point in a variety of cellular signaling cascades. The established involvement of mTOR activity in the cellular processes that contribute to the development and progression of cancer has identified mTOR as a major link in tumorigenesis.

Consequently, inhibitors of mTOR, have been developed and assessed for their safety and efficacy in patients with cancer [83].

*Everolimus RAD001 AFINITOR ®

Everolimus is an oral rapamycin compound targeting and inhibiting the PI3K/Akt/mTOR pathway a central regulator of cell growth, proliferation, survival, and angiogenesis. It is currently indicated in second line treatment of metastatic renal cell carcinoma after failure of one tyrosine kinase inhibitor. The RAD001 was tested at a dose of 10 mg daily in 2 phase II trials in second line treatment. The results of these 2 trials were presented this year at ASCO 2011 and showed limited activity of Everolimus (PR = 8%; PFS = 3.3 months; OS = 10.5 months, in one study) [84].

4. Histone Deacetylase Inhibitors

Histone deacetylases (HDACs) can regulate expression of tumor suppressor genes and activities of transcriptional factors involved in both cancer initiation and progression through alteration of either DNA or the structural components of chromatin. Recently, the role of gene repression through modulation such as acetylation in cancer patients has been clinically validated with several inhibitors of HDACs. In bladder cancer, Belinostat (PXD101) a HDACs inhibitor, was shown to be active according to several pre-clinical studies [85,86].

V. Chemotherapy in Muscle Invasive non Metastatic Disease (T2-T3-T4)

A. Rationale of Perioperative Chemotherapy

Even after radical surgery, half of the patients with tumors infiltrating the muscle develop distant metastasis and die of the disease. The benefit obtained in ORR, especially in complete response to chemotherapy, in metastatic setting leads to assess the role of perioperative chemotherapy in invasive tumors. Perioperative chemotherapy may be administered either before (neoadjuvant) or after (adjuvant) surgery in order to improve patient survival.

B. Neoadjuvant Chemotherapy

Neoadjuvant chemotherapy has been evaluated in several phase III trials in patients with stage T2–T4a bladder cancer (Table 1) [89–98] and in a meta-analysis [99]. Neoadjuvant chemotherapy has four theoretical advantages:

- the early treatment of micrometastatic disease,
- the systemic treatment is better tolerated by allowing the preoperative administration of chemotherapy drugs in optimal doses with less toxicity,
- the evaluation of chemo-sensitivity of the tumor,
- downstaging, which facilitates the surgical techniques.

The main inconvenient to primary chemotherapy is the delayed radical treatment (surgery or radiotherapy) in progressive patients. Two phase III trials and one meta-analysis confirmed the advantage of chemotherapy in neoadjuvant setting. The first study was conducted by the US Intergroup and concerned a randomized group of 317 patients with T2–T4a bladder cancer to surgery alone or to three cycles of MVAC chemotherapy followed by surgery [97]. The use of neoadjuvant chemotherapy is associated with a significant increase of pathological CRR (38% vs. 15%, p=0.001). At a median follow-up of 8.7 years, median survival (77 months vs. 46 months, p = 0.06) and 5-year survival (57% vs. 43%, p = 0.06) were significantly better in the MVAC arm. Although, one-third of patients treated with MVAC have developed high grade 3–4 toxicity, either hematologic or gastrointestinal. No toxic death was noted, and neoadjuvant chemotherapy had no negative impact on surgery or postoperative complications. The second phase III study conducted by the EORTC group concerned a randomized 976 patients having similar inclusion criteria between radical treatment alone (surgery or radiotherapy) or in combination with 3 cycles of neoadjuvant CMV (cisplatin, methotrexate, and vinblastine) chemotherapy [96]. Absolute improvement in time to progression at 3 years of 8.8% and 3-year survival of 5.5% (hazard ratio [HR] = 0.85, 95% CI, 0.71–1.02) for the chemotherapy arm has been reported [96]. Recently, the survival benefit was confirmed at 8-year followup (HR, 0.84; 95% CI, 0.72–0.99; p = 0.037, corresponding to an increase in 10-year survival from 30 to 36%) [100]. This study confirms statistically the significant benefit of chemotherapy in survival and local control. A meta-analysis of the ABC group has confirmed the benefit of neoadjuvant chemotherapy in muscle invasive tumors (cT2) [99]. The investigators have examined the individual data of more than 3,000 patients treated with neoadjuvant chemotherapy with cisplatin as part of 11 randomized trials. This meta-analysis showed a significant improvement in survival with a reduction in risk of death of 14% and an absolute benefit at 5 years estimated at 5% (p = 0.003). Moreover, this study showed that neoadjuvant chemotherapy can also reduce the risk of relapse by 22% with an absolute benefit of 9% at 5 years [99]. Based on these extended data, neoadjuvant chemotherapy is considered as the standard treatment in many institutions in the world (Americans and Europeans).

C. Adjuvant Chemotherapy

No clear evidence defines the role of adjuvant chemotherapy after primary surgery of invasive bladder cancer. The randomized studies published up to now have small size and do not clearly confirm the survival benefit of adjuvant chemotherapy in stage pT2 bladder cancer. The literature reports eight randomized trials with contradictory results [101–110]. In favor of adjuvant chemotherapy, only three studies showed a survival benefit [102–104, 110].

A meta-analysis of the ABC group based on individual data of 500 patients treated in 6 randomized trials demonstrated that adjuvant chemotherapy with cisplatin reduced the risk of death by 25% with an absolute benefit in survival of 9% at 3 years [111]. Recently, another positive phase III trial, was presented at ASCO annual meeting conducted by the Spanish group and included patients with stage pT3–pT4 tumor/N+ that were randomized to receive adjuvant chemotherapy based on cisplatin, gemcitabine and paclitaxel or observation. Unfortunately, this trial was interrupted early because of a lack of recruitment (n = 142) and higher hematologic toxicity of chemotherapy (9% of febrile neutropenia and 1 toxic death)

[110]. On the other hand, two published randomized trials including mainly patients with good prognosis showed no survival benefit with adjuvant chemotherapy [105, 106]. Similarly, preliminary results of an Italian multicenter randomized phase III trial included patients (n = 194) with stage pT2G3/pT3-4/N0-2 bladder cancer presented at ASCO 2008 showed no advantage on OS nor on PFS to favor the four cycles of GC chemotherapy [109]. Currently, the adjuvant chemotherapy with cisplatin based regimen is only an option in the case of lymph node involvement. Other trials are needed to confirm the role of chemotherapy in adjuvant setting.

Table 7. Randomized trials investigating neoadjuvant chemotherapy in invasive bladder cancer

Organization (year)	N	Primary end point	Treatments	Advantage in OS (primary end point)
Australia and England (1991) [89]	255	OS	CDDP → RT vs RT	No
CUETO/Spain (1995) [90]	121	OS	CDDP → Cyst vs Cyst	No
Italy (1995) [91]	104	OS	CDDP-5FU → Cyst vs Cyst	No
NCIC (1996) [92]	99	OS and local control	CDDP → RT or RT + Cyst vs RT or RT + Cyst	No
Nordic cystectomy trial 1 (1996) [93]	325	OS	CDDP-A → RT/Cyst vs RT + Cyst	No (advantage in stages T3/T4a)
G.U.O.N.E/Italy (1996) [94]	206	OS	MVAC → Cyst vs Cyst	No
G.I.S.T.V (1996) [95]	171	OS	MVEC → Cyst vs Cyst	No
MRC/EORTC (1999) [96]	976	OS	CMV → RT or Cyst or RT + Cyst vs RT or Cyst or RT + Cyst	Yes
SWOG (INT-0080) (2003) [97]	317	OS	MVAC → Cyst vs Cyst	Yes
Nordic cystectomy trial 2 (2002) [98]	317	OS	CDDP-M → Cyst vs Cyst	No

OS : Overall Survival, DFS : Disease free survival, ORR : Overall Response Rate, 5-FU : 5-fluorouracile, A : doxorubicin, MCAVI : methotrexate, carboplatin, and vinblastine, CMV : cisplatin, methotrexate, and vinblastine, CUETO : Club Urologico Espanol de Tratamiento Oncologico, Cyst : cystectomy, CDDP : cisplatin, EORTC : European Organization for Research and Treatment of Cancer, GISTV : Gruppo Italiano per lo Studio dei Tumori della Viscica (Italian Bladder Cancer Study Group), GUONE : Gruppo Uro-Oncologico del Nord Est (Northeast Uro-oncological Group), MRC : Medical Research Council, M : methotrexate; MVAC : methotrexate, vinblastine, doxorubicin, and cisplatin; M-VEC : methotrexate, vinblastine, epirubicin, et cisplatin, NCIC : National Cancer Institute of Canada, RT : rdiotherapy, SWOG : Southwest Oncology Group.

VI. Treatment Recommendations (Figure 1)

A. Metastatic Disease

1. First Line Treatment

In metastatic setting, chemotherapy based on cisplatin should be considered as standard treatment of choice for patients with good performance status (0-1) and good renal function-Glomerular filtration rate (GFR) > 60 mL/min. MVAC, HD-MVAC, gemcitabine-cisplatin and dose-dense gemcitabine-cisplatin should be considered as four standard first-line chemotherapy treatments for metastatic bladder TCC. Taxane-based doublets are inferior to the standard MVAC and should not be used in first-line. Carboplatin-based combinations are inferior to cisplatin based regimens and should be only used in unfit patients. The platinum-free doublets are efficient and should be evaluated in randomized phase III trials. The triplet combinations are more toxic but not more effective, and should not be used in practice. The sequential protocols are more toxic but not more effective and should be evaluated in randomized phase III trials. The role of targeted therapies in the management of metastatic bladder TCC has not yet been defined. Nevertheless, targeting angiogenesis seem to be very promising.

2. Second and Third Line Treatments

For patients with platinum sensitive disease, a second line treatment based on cisplatin should be used in patient eligible to cisplatin. For cisplatin ineligible patients, a regimens based on carboplatin can be used. Vinflunine and gemcitabine-paclitaxel are 2 reasonable therapeutic options in patients with cisplatin refractory disease. All active drugs can be used in second and third line treatments.

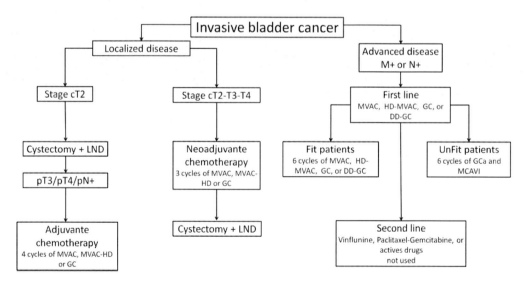

Figure 1. Treatment recommendations. LND: lymph node dissection.

B. Localized Disease

The evidence in 2011 (NCCN Guidelines, 2011 and EAU Guidelines, 2011) [112]

Neoadjuvant chemotherapy using three cycles of cisplatin based chemotherapy (MVAC, MVAC-HD or GC) is considered as a standard treatment in stages pT2–pT4 tumors.

It should be indicated in patients with good performance status (0–1) and good renal function glomerular filtration rate (GFR) [60 mL/min]. Adjuvant treatment based on four cycles of cisplatin based chemotherapy (MVAC, MVAC-HD or GC) is widely used in stages pT3–pT4/pN+ bladder cancer.

Conclusion

Chemotherapy plays a major role in the management of bladder cancer [87,88]. In the metastatic setting, palliative chemotherapy based on cisplatin type MVAC, HD-MVAC, or GC or DD-GC remains the treatment of choice. In unfit patients, Carboplatin based chemotherapy type Gemcitabin-Carboplatin or Methotrexate-Carboplatin-Vinblatine (MCAVI) is a good option for these patients. Radical cystectomy with pelvic lymph nodes dissection is the standard treatment of invasive transitional cell carcinoma of the bladder. Neoadjuvant chemotherapy is recognized by the scientific community as a standard treatment for stages T2–T4 disease [112]. In case of lymph node involvement, adjuvant chemotherapy should be considered as a treatment option. Novel therapies, targeting angiogenesis, have been shown to be very promising. Therapeutic investigations should be continued with the development of new drugs and targeted therapies to improve treatment results in the metastatic bladder cancer.

References

[1]   A. Jemal, F. Bray, M. M. Center, J. Ferlay, E. Ward, *CA. Cancer. J. Clin.* 61, 69 (2011).

[2]   Rathkopf D, Scher HI: Multidisciplinary Management of Genitourinary Malignancies in Malcolm R. Alison, editor. The cancer handbook. 2 edition. London: Jon Wiley & Son; 2007, 1432-52.

[3]   H. Wallerand, *Prog. Urol.* 19, 868 (2009).

[4]   N. Ismaili, S. Arifi, A. Flechon, O. El Mesbahi, J. Y. Blay, J. P. Droz, et al., *Bull. Cancer.* 96, E30 (2009).

[5]   D. F. Bajorin, P. M. Dodd, M. Mazumdar, M. Fazzari, J. A. McCaffrey, H. I. Scher, et al., *J. Clin. Oncol.* 17, 3173 (1999).

[6]   J. Bellmunt, T. K. Choueiri, R. Fougeray, F. A. Schutz, Y. Salhi, E. Winquist, S. Culine, H. von der Maase, D. J. Vaughn, J. E. Rosenberg, *J. Clin. Oncol.* 28, 1850 (2010).

[7]   R. Gagliano, H. Levin, M. N. El-Bolkainy, H. E. Wilson, R. L. Stephens, W. S. Fletcher, et al., *Am. J. Clin. Oncol.* 6, 215 (1983).

[8]   M. S. Soloway, A. Einstein, M. P. Corder, W. Bonney, G. R. Prout, J. Coombs, *Cancer*
      1983, 52(5):767-72.

[9]   W. G. Harke, F. J. Meyers, F. S. Freiha, J. M. Palmer, L. D. Shortliffe, J. F. Hannigan,
      et al., *J. Clinl. Oncol.* 1463 (1985).

[10] M. Troner, R. Birch, G. A. Omura, S. Williams, *J. Urol.* 137, 660 (1987).

[11] C. N. Sternberg, A. Yagoda, H. I. Scher, R. C. Watson, T. Ahmed, L. R. Weiselberg, et
      al., *J. Urol.* 133, 403 (1985).

[12] C. N. Sternberg, *Crit. Rev. Oncol. Hematol.* 31, 193 (1999).

[13] C. J. Logothetis, F. H. Dexeus, L Finn, A. Sella, R. J. Amato, A. G. Ayala, et al., *J.
      Clin. Oncol.* 8, 1050 (1990).

[14] P. J. Loehrer, L. H. Einhorn, P. J. Elson, E. D. Crawford, P. Kuebler, I. Tannock, et al.,
      J. Clin. Oncol. 10, 1066 (1992).

[15] C. N. Sternberg, P. H. de Mulder, J. H. Schornagel, C. Théodore, S. D. Fossa, A. T. van
      Oosterom, et al., *J. Clin. Oncol.* 19, 2638 (2001).

[16] C. N. Sternberg, P. de Mulder, J. H. Schornagel, C. Theodore, S. D. Fossa, A. T. van
      Oosterom, et al., *Eur. J. Cancer.* 42, 50 (2006).

[17] J. Bellmunt, S. Albiol, A. R. de Olano, J. Pujadas, P. Maroto, *Ann. Oncol.* 17:113
      (2006).

[18] H. von der Maase, S. W. Hansen, J. T. Roberts, L. Dogliotti, T. Oliver, M. J. Moore, I.
      Bodrogi, P. Albers, A. Knuth, C. M. Lippert, P. Kerbra, P. Sanchez Rovira, P. Wersall,
      S. P. Cleall, D. F. Roychowdhury, I. Tomlin, C. M. Visseren-Grul, P. F. Conte, *J. Clin.
      Oncol.* 18, 3068 (2000).

[19] H. von der Maas, L. Sengelov, J. T. Roberts, S. Ricci, L. Dogliotti, T. Oliver, et al., *J.
      Clin. Oncol.* 4602 (2005).

[20] A. Bamias, A. Karadimou, S. Lampaki, G. Aravantinos, I. Xanthakis, C. Papandreou, et
      al., *J. Clin. Oncol.* 29 (suppl; abstr 4510) (2011).

[21] P. A. Burch, R. L. Richardson, S. S. Cha, D. J. Sargent, H. C. Pitot, J. S. Kaur, et al., *J.
      Urol.* 164, 1538 (2000).

[22] R. Dreicer, J. Manola, B. J. Roth, M. B. Cohen, A. K. Hatfield, G. Wilding, *J. Clin.
      Oncol.,* 18, 1058 (2000).

[23] M. A. Dimopoulos, C. Bakoyannis, V. Georgoulias, C. Papadimitriou, L. A.
      Moulopoulos, C. Deliveliotis, et al., Ann. Oncol. 10, 1385 (1999).

[24]. X. Garcia del Muro, E. Marcuello, J. Gumá, L. Paz-Ares, M. A. Climent, J. Carles, et
      al., *Br. J. Cancer.* 86, 326 (2002).

[25] L. Sengelov, C. Kamby, B. Lund, S. A. Engelholm, *J. Clin. Oncol.*16, 3392 (1998).

[26] A. Bamias, G. Aravantinos, C. Deliveliotis, D. Bafaloukos, C. Kalofonos, N. Xiros, et
      al., *J. Clin. Oncol.* 22, 220 (2004).

[27] J. Waxman, C. Barton. *Cancer. Treat. Rev.* 19, 21(1993).

[28] B.G. Redman, D. C. Smith, L. Flaherty, W. Du, M. Hussain, *J. Clin. Oncol.* 16:184
      (1998).

[29] E. J. Small, D. Lew, B. G. Redman, D. P. Petrylak, N. Hammond, H. M. Gross, et al., *J.
      Clin. Oncol.* 2000, 18, 2537 (2000).

[30] D. J. Vaughn, S. B. Malkowicz, B. Zoltick, R. Mick, P. Ramchandani, C. Holroyde, et
      al.: Paclitaxel plus carboplatin in advanced carcinoma of the urothelium: an active and
      tolerable outpatient regimen. *J Clin Oncol* 1998, 16:255-60.

[31] R. Dreicer, J. Manola, B. J. Roth, W. A. See, S. Kuross, M. J. Edelman, G. R. Hudes, G. Wilding, *Cancer*. 100, 1639 (2004).

[32] J. Bellmunt, R. de Wit, J. Albanell, J. Baselga, *Eur. J. Cancer*. 37, 2212 (2001).

[33] M. Nogué-Aliguer, J. Carles, A. Arrivi, O. Juan, L. Alonso, A. Font, et al., Cancer. 97, 2180 (2003).

[34] C. Shannon, C. Crombie, A. Brooks, H. Lau, M. Drummond, H. Gurney, *Ann. Oncol.* 12, 947 (2001).

[35] L. Dogliotti, G. Cartenì, S. Siena, O. Bertetto, A. Martoni, A. Bono, et al., *Eur. Urol.* 52, 134 (2007).

[36] E. Winquist, E. Vokes, M. J. Moore, L. P. Schumm, K. Hoving, W. M; Stadler, Urol. Oncol. 23, 150 (2005).

[37] M. De Santis, J. Bellmunt, G. Mead, J. M. Kerst, M. G. Leahy, G. Daugaard, et al., J. Clin. Oncol. 28, 18s, abstract LBA4519 (2010).

[38] D. S. Kaufman, M. A. Carducci, T. M. Kuzel, M. B. Todd, W. K. Oh, M. R. Smith, et al., *Urol. Oncol.* 22, 393 (2004).

[39] J. Li, B. Juliar, C. Yiannoutsos, R. Ansari, E. Fox, M. J. Fisch, et al., *J. Clin. Oncol.* 23, 1185 (2005).

[40] A. A. Meluch, F. A. Greco, H. A. Burris, T. O'Rourke, G. Ortega, R. G. Steis, et al., J. Clin. Oncol. 19, 3018 (2001).

[41] D. S. Kaufman, M. A. Carducci, T. M. Kuzel, M. B. Todd, W. K. Oh, M. R. Smith, et al., *Urol. Oncol.* 22, 393 (2004).

[42] A. Ardavanis, D. Tryfonopoulos, A. Alexopoulos, C. Kandylis, G. Lainakis, G. Rigatos, *Br. J. Cancer*. 92, 645 (2005).

[43] H. Dumez, M. Martens, J. Selleslach, G. Guetens, G. De Boeck, R. Aerts, et al., *Anticancer. Drugs*. 18, 211 (2007).

[44] B. J. Gitlitz, C. Baker, Y. Chapman, H. J. Allen, L. D. Bosserman, R. Patel, et al., *Cancer*. 98, 1863 (2003).

[45] S. Li, R. Dreicer, B. Roth, J. Manoloa, M. Cooney, G. Wilding, *J. Clin. Oncol.* 25, abstract 5079 (2007).

[46] H. von der Maase, J. Lehmann, G. Gravis, H. Joensuu, P. F. Geertsen, J. Gough, et al., *Ann. Oncol.* 17, 1533 (2006).

[47] J. Bellmunt, V. Guillem, L. Paz-Ares, J. L. González-Larriba, J. Carles, E. Batiste-Alentorn, et al., *J. Clin. Oncol.* 18, 3247 (2000).

[48] J. Bellmunt, H. von der Maase, G. M. Mead, J. Heyer, N. Houede, L. G. Paz-Ares, et al., *J. Clin. Oncol.* 25, abstract LBA5030 (2007).

[49] D. F. Bajorin, J. A. McCaffrey, P. M. Dodd, S. Hilton, M. Mazumdar, W. K. Kelly, et al., *Cancer*. 88, 1671 (2000).

[50] M. Hussain, U. Vaishampayan, W. Du, B. Redman, D. C. Smith, *J. Clin. Oncol.* 19, 2527 (2001).

[51] J. D. Hainsworth, A. A. Meluch, S. Litchy, F. M. Schnell, J. D. Bearden, K. Yost, et al., *Cancer*. 103, 2298 (2005).

[52] M. J. Edelman, F. J. Meyers, T. R. Miller, S. G. William, R. Gandour Edwards, R. De Vere white, *Urology*. 55, 521 (2000).

[53] S. M. Tu, E. Hossan, R. Amato, R. Kilbourn, Logothesis, *J. Urol.* 154, 1719 (1995).

[54] L. Y. Law, P. N. Lara, F. J. Meyers, N. A. Dawson, M. J. Edelman, *J. Clin. Oncol.* 20, abstract 767 (2001).

[55] D. Pectasides, A. Visvikis, A. Aspropotamitis, A. Halikia, N. Karvounis, M. Dimitriadis, et al., *Eur. J. Cancer.* 36, 74 (2000).

[56] M. I. Milowsky, D. M. Nanus, F. C. Maluf, S. Mironov, W. Shi, A. Iasonos, J. Riches, A. Regazzi, D. F. Bajorin, J. Clin. Oncol. 27, 4062 (2009).

[57] M. D. Galsky, A. Iasonos, S. Mironov, J. Scattergood, M. G. Boyle, D. F. Bajorin, *Cancer.* 109, 549 (2007).

[58] G. Di Lorenzo, R. Autorino, A. Giordano, M. Giuliano, M. D'Armiento, A. R. Bianco, et al., Jpn. J. Clin. Oncol. 34, 747 (2004).

[59] M. Khorsand, J. Lange, L. Feun, N. J. Clendeninn, M. Collier, G. Wilding, *Invest. New. Drugs.* 15, 157 (1997).

[60] C. J. Sweeney, B. J. Roth, F. F. Kabbinavar, D. J. Vaughn, M. Arning, R. E. Curiel, et al., J. Clin. Oncol. 24, 3451 (2006).

[61] Y. R. Seo, S. H. Kim, H. J. Kim, C. K. Kim, S. K. Park, E. S. Koh, D. S. Hong, J. *Hematol. Oncol.* 3, 4 (2010).

[62] J. Bellmunt, C. Théodore, T. Demkov, B. Komyakov, L. Sengelov, G. Daugaard, et al., *J. Clin. Oncol.* 27, 4454 (2009).

[63] P. Albers, S. I. Park, G. Niegisch, G. Fechner, U. Steiner, J. Lehmann, D. Heimbach, A. Heidenreich, R. Fimmers, R. Siener, *Ann. Oncol.* 22, 288 (2010).

[64] D. I. Quinn, A. Aparicio, D. D. Tsao-Wei, S. G. Groshen, T. B. Dorff, T. W. Synold, et al., *J. Clin. Oncol.* 28, abstract 4539 (2010).

[65] [http://www.clinicaltrials.gov/ct2/results?term=%22bladder+cancer%22+metastatic +disease].

[66] N. M. Hahn, W. M. Stadler, R. T. Zon, D. M. Waterhouse, J. Picus, S. R. Nattam, et al., *J. Clin. Oncol.* 28, abstract 4541 (2010).

[67] D. J. Gallagher, M. I. Milowsky, S. R. Gerst, N. Ishill, J. Riches, A. Regazzi, et al., *J. Clin. Oncol.* 28, 1373 (2010).

[68] D. J. Gallagher, M. I. Milowsky, S. R. Gerst, S. Tickoo, N. Ishill, A. Regazzi, et al., *J. Clin. Oncol.* 27, abstract 5072 (2009).

[69] D. Bradley, S. Daignault, D. C. Smith, D. Nanus, S. Tagawa, W. M. Stadler, et al., *J. Clin. Oncol.* 27, abstract 5073 (2009).

[70] M. D. Galsky, G. Sonpavde, B. A. Hellerstedt, S. A. McKenney, T. E. Hutson, M. A. Rauch, et al., *J. Clin. Oncol.* 28, abstract 4573 (2010).

[71] J. Bellmunt, J. L. Gonzalez-Larriba, J. P. Maroto, J. Carles, D. E. Castellano, B. Mellado, et al., *J. Clin. Oncol.* 28, abstract 4540 (2010).

[72] R. Dreicer, H. Li, M. N. Stein, R. P. DiPaola, M. Eleff, B. J. Roth, et al., *J. Clin. Oncol.* 26, abstract 5083 (2008).

[73] S. Krege, H. Rexer, F. vom Dorp, P. Albers, P. De Geeter, T. Klotz, *J. Clin. Oncol.* 28, abstract 4574 (2010).

[74] M. I. Milowsky, G. L. Carlson, M. M. Shi, G. Urbanowitz, Y. Zhang, C. N Sternberg, J. Clin. Oncol. 29, abstract TPS186 (2011).

[75] U. Lönn, S. Lönn, S. Friberg, B. Nilsson, C. Silfverswärd, B. Stenkvist, *Clin. Cancer. Res.* 1, 1189 (1995).

[76] R. T. Vollmer, P. A. Humphrey, P. E. Swanson, M. R. Wick, M. L. Hudson, *Cancer.* 82, 715 (1998).

[77] R. E. Jimenez, M. Hussain, F. J. Bianco, U. Vaishampayan, P. Tabazcka, W. A. Sakr, et al., *Clin. Cancer. Res.* 7, 2440 (2001).

[78] G. De Pinieux, D. Colin, A. Vincent-Salomon, J. Couturier, D. Amsellem-Ouazana, P. Beuzeboc, et al., *Virchows. Arch.* 444, 415 (2004).

[79] M. H. Hussain, G. R. MacVicar, D. P. Petrylak, R. L. Dunn, U. Vaishampayan, P. N. Lara, et al., *J. Clin. Oncol.* 25, 2218 (2007).

[80] D. Petrylak, J. R. Faulkner, P. J. Van Veldhuizen, M. Mansukhani, E. D. Crawford, *J. Clin. Oncol.* 22, abstract 1619 (2003).

[81] G. K. Philips, S. Halabi, B. L. Sanford, D. Bajorin, E. J. Small, *Ann. Oncol.* 20, 1074 (2009).

[82] C. Wülfing, J. P. Machiels, D. J. Richel, M. O. Grimm, U. Treiber, M. R. De Groot, et al., *Cancer.* 115, 2881 (2009).

[83] N. Ismaili, M. Amzerin, A. Flechon. *J. Hematol. Oncol.* 4, 35 (2011).

[84] M. I. Milowsky, A. Trout, A. M. Regazzi, I. Garcia-Grossman, A. Flaherty, S. Tickoo, et al., *J. Clin. Oncol.* 28, abstract TPS229 (2010).

[85] Tan J, Cang S, Ma Y, Petrillo RL, Liu D: Novel histone deacetylase inhibitors in clinical trials as anti-cancer agents. J Hematol Oncol 2010, 3:5.

[86] X. S. Xu, L. Wang, J. Abrams, G. Wang, *J. Hematol. Oncol.* 4, 17 (2011).

[87] N. Ismaili, M. Amzerin, S. Elmajjaoui, J. P. Droz, A. Flechon, H. Errihani, *Prog. Urol.* 21, 369 (2011).

[88] N. Ismaili, S. Elmajjaoui, Y. Bensouda, R. Belbaraka, H. Abahssain, W. Allam, et al., Oncol. Rev. (2011).

[89] Wallace DM, Raghavan D, Kelly KA, Sandeman TF, Conn IG, Teriana N et al., *Br. J. Urol.* 67, 608 (1991).

[90] J. A. Martinez-Pineiro, M. Gonzalez Martin, F. Arocena, N. Flores, C. R. Roncero, J. A. Portillo, A. Escudero, F. Jimenez Cruz, S. Isorna, *J. Urol.* 153, 964 (1995).

[91] M. Orsatti, A. Curotto, L. Canobbio, D. Guarneri, D. Scarpati, Venturini M et al., Alternating chemo-radiotherapy in bladder cancer: a conservative approach. *Int. J. Radiat. Oncol. Biol. Phys.* 33, 173 (1995).

[92] C. M. Coppin, M. K. Gospodarowicz, K. James, I. F. Tannock, B. Zee, J. Carson et al., *J. Clin. Oncol.* 14, 2901 (1996).

[93] P. U. Malmstro¨m, E. Rintala, R. Wahlqvist, P. Hellstro¨m, S. Hellsten, E. Hannisdal, *J. Urol.* 155, 1903 (1996).

[94] P. Bassi, F. Pagano, G. Pappagallo, *Eur. Urol.* 33, abstract 567 (1998).

[95] GISTV (Italian Bladder Cancer Study Group), *J. Chemother.* 8,345 (1996).

[96] *Lancet.* 354, 533 (1999).

[97] H. B. Grossman, R. B. Natale, C. M. Tangen, V. O. Speights, N. J. Vogelzang, D. L. Trump et al., *N. Engl. J. Med.* 349, 859 (2003).

[98] A. Sherif, E. Rintala, O. Mestad, J. Nilsson, L. Holmberg, S. Nilsson, P. U. Malmstro¨m, *Scand. J. Urol. Nephrol.* 36, 419 (2002).

[99] Advanced Bladder Cancer (ABC) Meta-analysis Collaboration. *Eur. Urol.* 48, 189 (2005).

[100] G. Griffiths, R. Hall, R. Sylvester, D. Raghavan, M. K. Parmar International phase III trial assessing neoadjuvant cisplatin, methotrexate, and vinblastine chemotherapy for muscle-invasive bladder cancer: long-term results of the BA06 30894 trial. *J. Clin. Oncol.* 29(16):2171 (2011).

[101] C. J. Logothetis, D. E. Johnson, C. Chong, F. H. Dexeus, A. Sella, S. Ogden et al., *J. Clin. Oncol.* 6, 1590 (1988).

[102] D. G. Skinner, J. R. Daniels, C. A. Russell, G. Lieskovsky, S. D. Boyd, P. Nichols et al., The role of adjuvant chemotherapy following cystectomy for invasive bladder cancer: a prospective comparative trial. *J. Urol.* 145, 459 (1991).

[103] M. Sto¨ckle, W. Meyenburg, S. Wellek, G. Voges, U. Gertenbach, J. W. Thu¨roff et al., *J. Urol.* 148, 302 (1992).

[104] M. Sto¨ckle, W. Meyenburg, S. Wellek, G. E. Voges, M. Rossmann, U. Gertenbach et al., *J Urol* 153(1):47 (1995).

[105] U. E. Studer, M. Bacchi, C. Biedermann, P. Jaeger, R. Kraft, L. Mazzucchelli et al., *J. Urol.* 152, 81(1994).

[106] A. V. Bono, C. Benvenuti, A. Gibba, *Acta. Urol. Ital.* 11, 5(1997).

[107] F. Freiha, J. Reese, F. M. A. Torti. *J. Urol.* 155, 495 (1996).

[108] T. Otto, C. Bo¨rgemann, S. Krege, *Eur. Urol.* 39, 147(2001).

[109] F. Cognetti, E. M. Ruggeri, A. Felici, M. Gallucci, G. Muto, C. F. Pollera, et al.. *J. Clin. Oncol.* 26, abstract 5023 (2008).

[110] L. G. Paz-Ares, E. Solsona, E. Esteban, A. Saez, J. Gonzalez-Larriba, A. Anton, et al., *J. Clin. Oncol.* 28, abstract LBA4518 (2010).

[111] Advanced Bladder Cancer (ABC) Meta-analysis Collaboration, *Eur. Urol.* 48, 202 (2005).

[112] A. Stenzl, N. C. Cowan, M. de Santis, M. A. Kuczyk, A. S. Merseburger, M. J. Ribal et al., Treatment of muscle-invasive and metastatic bladder cancer: update of the EAU guidelines. *Eur. Urol.* 59, 1009 (2011).

In: Handbook of Genitourinary Medicine: New Research   ISBN: 978-1-62618-226-4
Editor: Rashmi R. Singh   © 2013 Nova Science Publishers, Inc.

Chapter VIII

The Genetics of Pediatric Nephrotic Syndrome

*Aiysha Abid**

Centre for Human Genetics and Molecular Medicine,
Sindh Institute of Urology and Transplantation, Karachi, Pakistan

Abstract

The glomerular filtration barrier (GFB) in the kidney plays a central role in the ultrafiltration of plasma. Certain inherited or acquired defects in the structure and function of this barrier result in the urinary loss of proteins that ultimately cause nephrotic syndrome (NS). It is the most common kidney disease found in children. Depending on the age at disease presentation, pediatric NS can be classified clinically as congenital (CNS), infantile and childhood onset. Most of the patients respond well to initial steroid therapy and show a favorable long term renal outcome. However, a small proportion show resistance to steroid therapy and are referred to as steroid resistant nephrotic syndrome (SRNS). Such patients often have a genetic component with a poor renal outcome and tend to progress rapidly to renal failure. Disease-causing mutations in several genes that are highly expressed in the GFB and podocytes have been reported to cause pediatric NS. Mutations in different genes show variability in the clinical course and severity of disease progression as well as treatment options. This chapter presents an overview of the current advances in the genetic basis of NS and associated gene mutations.

Introduction

The glomerular filtration barrier (GFB) in the kidney is responsible for the outflow of solutes from the blood capillaries to the urinary space. It consists of three layers: the

---

* Email: aiyshaabid@gmail.com.

endothelium, the glomerular basement membrane (GBM) and the podocytes. The endothelial cell layer separates the blood and tissue compartments and is surrounded by the GBM. The GBM is a thick basement membrane and is rich in the negatively charged glycosaminoglycans that are responsible for repelling proteins from the blood by electrostatic forces during the process of filtration. The podocytes, or visceral epithelial cells, line the outer surface of the GBM. They have highly specialized actin-based cytoplasmic extensions called the foot processes [1]. Podocytes are the first cells to be differentiated during renal glomerular development forming a disk-like layer of epithelial cells. During the maturation process, they lose their pluripotency and proliferative ability and develop their interdigitating foot processes that are crucial for the formation of early cell-cell contact.

The structural architecture of these foot processes is the actin-based cytoskeleton that forms a firm but highly dynamic structure. The interdigitating foot processes of adjacent podocytes form pores of about 40 nm in width called the slit diaphragm (SD). The SD forms a "zipper-like" cell-cell contact between the podocytes. It is a sophisticated multi-protein complex that maintains the foot process architecture and controls the ultra-filtration of molecules via signalling to the actin cytoskeleton of the podocyte. The podocytes, with their highly dynamic foot processes, and the slit diaphragm together form the central structure for the barrier function of the glomerulus. They also produce the extra-cellular matrix proteins that are responsible for the maintenance of the GBM. They provide mechanical support for the glomerular capillary wall. During the filtration process, the GFB is responsible for the selective permeability of molecules based upon their size and charge. It selectively permits ultra filtration of water and solutes and is responsible for the production of 130-180 l of ultrafiltrate that is free of macromolecules that are >40 KDa such as albumins and clotting factors etc. Any structural or functional disruption of this barrier increases the permeability of macromolecules leading to the clinical presentation of nephrotic syndrome [2].

Nephrotic Syndrome

Nephrotic syndrome is the most common type of kidney disease found in children. It is characterized by massive proteinuria, hypoalbuminemia and edema. The children generally show periorbital swelling with or without generalized edema. Pediatric NS can be classified on the basis of age at presentation as congenital (CNS), infantile and childhood onset. CNS appears quite early, in utero or during the first three months of life. Infantile and childhood onset NS is diagnosed during and after the first year of life respectively. However, in the last two decades, the identification of the genetic causes has modified the clinical classification of NS.

The exact pathogenesis of NS in children is not well established. Clinically, NS is responsive to corticosteroid therapy and the clinical course can be characterized by remission or relapse of the proteinuria. It has been estimated that more than 80% of the children with idiopathic nephrotic syndrome respond to steroid treatment with the resolution of proteinuria and edema. Thus the condition is referred to as the steroid-sensitive nephrotic system (SSNS). Patients often show a favorable long term renal outcome but are at risk of morbidity from episodes of relapses and long term corticosteroid exposure. Around 10-20% of the patients fail to enter remission usually after 4-8 weeks of corticosteroid treatment and are labeled as steroid-resistant nephrotic syndrome (SRNS) [3]. The patients with SRNS are also at increased risk of developing renal complications such as chronic kidney disease (CKD) or end stage renal disease (ESRD) due to the progressive damage of the GFB. Corticosteroid treatment in these patients increases the risk of ESRD for more than 50% within 4 years of the diagnosis of SRNS [4]. Corticosteroid therapy has been established as a standard therapy for the last 50 years but neither the target cells nor the mechanism of action of these agents has been clearly determined in NS [5].

With respect to response to corticosteroid therapy and renal survival, the clinical course of the disease in patients with hereditary NS differs from patients with non-genetic disease. It is estimated that 71% of the patients with hereditary causes progress to ESRD in approximately 8 years of follow-up time as compared to the 29% cases with non hereditary SRNS [6]. In the last two decades, substantial progress has been made in the identification of the genetic basis of the hereditary forms of NS. Several genes have been identified that, when mutated, lead to the inherited forms of the disease. A large proportion of these genes are expressed specifically in the podocytes, highlighting the importance of these specialized cells as the site of cellular injury in NS. This chapter will describe the role of these genes and their protein products in the pathogenesis of NS.

Epidemiology

In the USA, the estimated annual incidence of pediatric NS is 2-7 cases per 100,000 children younger than 16 years of age with a cumulative frequency of 16 cases per 100,000 individuals [7]. In some populations, such as those of Finnish and Mennonite origin, the incidence of congenital NS is very high, about 1 case in 10,000 individuals and 1 in 500 births respectively [8, 9]. Similarly in New Zealand, the incidence is almost 20 cases per million children under 15 years of age [10]. Geographic or ethnic differences have also been reported to contribute towards the incidence of NS as Black and Hispanic children have an increased risk of SRNS and FSGS compared to American children [11, 12]. A 6-fold higher incidence of NS is also reported in the Asian populations compared to the European populations [13]. In contrast, data from Africa suggest that idiopathic NS is relatively less common among African children, where the glomerular lesions are commonly induced by infectious agents [14, 15]. The reported variations of geographic and ethnic distribution of NS underscore the genetic and environmental influences in the development of the disease [16]. In the occurrence of NS among young children, the males to females ratio is 2:1. However, this gender difference disappears among adolescent children and adults where the incidence is equal among the two sexes [7, 17].

Although the incidence of idiopathic nephrotic syndrome has been stable over the last 30 years, varying histopathological patterns are observed in different regions and populations of the world. According to "The International Study of Kidney Diseases in Children" (1978), the most common histologic correlate of childhood NS is sporadic MCNS (minimal change nephrotic syndrome) affecting 77% of the children, followed by FSGS (focal segmental glomerulosclerosis; 8%) [18]. However, some recent studies have shown a rise in the incidence of FSGS in the NS patients [19]. In renal biopsies, SRNS is associated with the histological features of FSGS in 75% of the cases, while 20% of the cases show MCNS [20].

According to the data from India and Pakistan, MCD and its variants are the leading causes of NS in children under 8 years of age followed by FSGS, which is the predominant pathology in SRNS and adolescent NS [21, 22].

Pathology

The appearance of massive proteinuria is the most common manifestation in all cases of NS. This may be a consequence of primary glomerular injury or immunological abnormality. Glomerular pathology in NS mostly appears as minimal change disease (MCD or MCNS), focal segmental glomerulosclerosis (FSGS) or diffuse mesengial sclerosis (DMS). MCNS is characterized by responsiveness to steroid treatment accompanied by more or less frequent relapses (Figure 1).

In light microscopy, the glomeruli appear normal, but electron microscopy usually shows epithelial changes with the loss of foot processes. Minor changes such as mild mesengial hypercellularity, mild mesengial thickening and focal glomerular obsolescence are also shown. FSGS is defined as the presence of sclerosis in a certain proportion of the glomeruli (focal) as well as certain parts of each affected glomerulus (segmental; Figure 2). With the progression of NS, the sclerosis expands and is converted into a more diffused and global pattern.

The effacement of foot processes of the podocytes is another common finding in FSGS. Corticosteroid treatment has been shown to induce remission in more than 90% of children with MCNS. By contrast, the majority of the children with FSGS do not respond to oral glucocorticoids [20, 23]. Therefore, renal biopsy is recommended in the SRNS children to identify patients with MCNS for whom a positive response to therapy can be achieved and to avoid side effects of long term therapy in the cases of steroid resistance [20].

The Genetics of Nephrotic Syndrome

The majority of early onset NS cases have a genetic origin with a widespread age of onset that ranges from fetal life to several years [24]. Congenital and infantile NS mostly have a genetic cause and may occur as an isolated kidney disease. However, some syndromic forms are also documented with extra renal manifestations such as Denys-Drash syndrome (DDS; OMIM # 194080), Frasier syndrome (FS; OMIM # 136680), Pierson syndrome (OMIM # 609049) and Galloway-Mowat syndrome (OMIM # 251300). NS can be caused by a variety of glomerular and systemic diseases, but the most common type in childhood is idiopathic nephrotic syndrome [25].

During the last two decades, mutations in several genes that are highly expressed in the GFB and podocytes have been reported to cause pediatric NS (Table 1). Most of these gene products are important components of the podocytes and SD. Among these, NPHS1, NPHS2, CD2AP, TRPC6 and ACTN4 are cytoskeletal proteins; LAMB2 is a component of the glomerular basement membrane; PLCE1 is involved in the podocyte signalling processes; WT1 and LMX1B are transcription factors that control gene regulation and podocyte differentiation and COQ6 resides in the mitochondria (Figure 3).

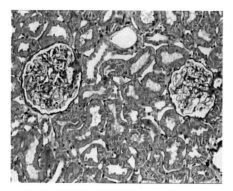

Figure 1. Low-power view showing two glomeruli and the surrounding tubules with minor changes in the glomeruli on light microscopy. The surrounding parenchyma is unremarkable, an essential feature supporting the diagnosis of minimal change disease. (PAS, ×100; courtesy Dr. Mohammad Mubarak).

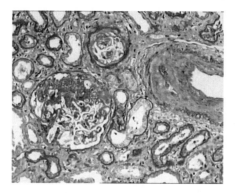

Figure 2. Medium-power view showing one intact glomerulus in the center of the field showing segmental sclerosis/hyalinosis involving the upper half of the glomerulus with adhesion formation with the Bowman's capsule, the cardinal features of diagnosis of FSGS. The lower half of the glomerulus is unremarkable. There is moderate fibrointimal thickening of part of wall of one interlobular size artery, tubular atrophy and interstitial inflammation (PAS, ×200; courtesy Dr. Mohammad Mubarak).

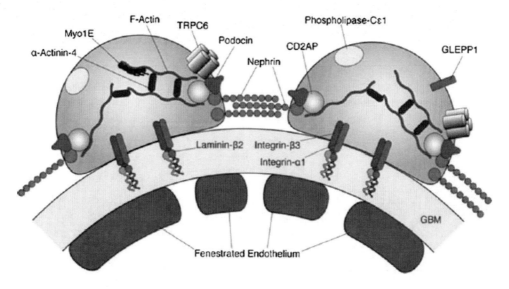

Figure 3. The podocytes and slit diaphragm with orchestrating proteins [26].

Table 1. List of genes and their respective phenotypes that are known to cause syndromic and isolated NS

Gene	protein	Location/function	Phenotype	Histology	Mode of Inheritance	Refere-nce
NPHS1	Nephrin	[a]SD, structural protein, podocyte signaling,	[b]CNS, [c]SRNS	[d]MCD, [e]FSGS, [f]MPGN	[g]AR	[27]
NPHS2	Podocin	SD, linked with nephrin, podocyte signaling	CNS, SRNS	FSGS	AR	[28]
WT1	[h]WT1 tumor suppressor	Nuclear transcription factor	[i]DDS, [j]FS, isolated SRNS	[k]DMS, FSGS	[l]AD/AR	[31, 66]
PLCE1	Phospholipase C ε 1	SD, podocyte signaling	DMS, SRNS	DMS, FSGS	AR incomplete penetrance	[52]
LAMB2	Laminin β2	[m]GBM, linkage between podocyte and GBM	Pierson's syndrome	FSGS, DMS	AR	[100]
ACTN4	Actinin 4	Podocyte actin regulating	SRNS adult onset	FSGS	AD	[81]
TRPC6	Transient receptor potential C6 ion channel	SD, cell signaling, mediate calcium influx	SRNS	FSGS	AD	[78]
INF2	Inverted formin 2	Podocyte actin regulating	SRNS, Charcot-Marie tooth disease	FSGS	AD	[87]
CD2AP	CD2 associated protein	SD, adapter protein,	SRNS	FSGS	AD/AR	[101]
PTPRO	Glomerular epithelial protein-1 GLEPP1	Podocyte foot processes, glomerular pressure regulation	SRNS	FSGS	AR	[92]
MYO1E	Nonmuscle class I myosin 1E (Myo1E)	plasma membrane, maintain podocyte structural integrity	SRNS	FSGS	AR	[93]
LMX1B	LIM homeobox transcription factor 1B	Nuclear transcription factor, podocyte differentiation	Nail-Patella syndrome	FSGS	AD incomplete penetrance	[102]
COQ6	Coenzyme Q10 biosynthesis monooxy-genase 6	Mitochondria	SRNS with sensori-neural deafness	FSGS	AR	[103]

[a] Slit diaphragm; [b]congenital nephrotic syndrome; [c]steroid resistant nephrotic syndrome; [d]minimal change disease; [e]focal segmental glomerulosclerosis; [f]mesengial proliferative glomerulonephritis; [g]autosomal recessive; [h]Wilms' tumor; [i]Denys-Drash syndrome; [j]Frasier syndrome; [k]diffuse mesangial sclerosis; [l]autosomal dominant; [m]glomerular basement membrane.

Table 2. Nephrotic syndrome and associated disorders as listed in the OMIM (http://www.ncbi.nlm.nih.gov/omim)

No.	OMIM ID	LOCUS	CYTOGENETIC LOCATION	GENE
1	256300	Nephrotic syndrome, type 1; NPHS1	19q13.12	*NPHS1*
2.	603278	Focal segmental glomerulosclerosis 1, FSGS1	19q13.2	*ACTN4*
3.	600995	Nephrotic syndrome, type 2, NPHS2	1q25.2	*NPHS2*
4.	610725	Nephrotic syndrome, type 3, NPHS3	10q23.33	*PLCE1*
5.	256370	Nephrotic syndrome, type 4; NPHS4	11p13	*WT1*
6.	603965	Focal segmental glomerulosclerosis 2; FSGS2	11q22.1	*TRPC6*
7.	614199	Nephrotic syndrome, type 5, with or without ocular abnormalities, NPHS5	3p21.31	*LAMB2*
8.	614196	Nephrotic syndrome, type 6, NPHS6	12p12.3	*PTPRO*
9.	613237	Focal segmental glomerulosclerosis 5, FSGS5	14q32.33	*INF2*
10.	607832	Focal segmental glomerulosclerosis 3, susceptibility to; FSGS3	6p12.3	*CD2AP*
11.	614131	Focal segmental glomerulosclerosis 6, FSGS6	15q22.2	*MYO1E*
12.	301050	Alport syndrome, x-linked; ATS	Xq22.3	*COL4A5*
13.	612551	Focal segmental glomerulosclerosis 4, susceptibility to; FSGS4	22q12.3	*APOL1*
14.	203780	Alport syndrome, autosomal recessive	2q36.3	*COL4A3*
15.	251300	Galloway-Mowat syndrome,	–	–
16.	614748	Interstitial lung disease, nephrotic syndrome, and epidermolysis bullosa, congenital	17p21.33	*ITGA3*
17.	607426	CoQ10 deficiency, primary, 1,	4q21.23	*COQ2*
18.	613606	Forsythe-wakeling syndrome; FWS,	1p33-p31.1	–
19.	614650	Coenzyme q10 deficiency, primary, 6; COQ10D6	14q24.3	*COQ6*
20.	254900	Action myoclonus-renal failure syndrome; AMRF	4q21.1	*SCARB2*
21.	161200	Nail-patella syndrome; NPS	9q33.3	*LMX1B*
22.	609469	Alport/focal segmental glomerulosclerosis-like syndrome	11q24	–

Mutations in any of the genes result in the disruption of the complex network of these proteins, foot process effacement and loss of SD [26]. As podocytes have been shown to be involved in GBM synthesis and fenestration of the endothelial cells, any injury to the podocyte not only affects the structure of the podocyte or SD alone, but also disintegrates the adjacent structures and consequently alters glomerular permeability.

Mutations in the *NPHS1*, *NPHS2* and *PLCE1* genes have been found in most of the severe cases of congenital and early onset NS whereas, mutations in the *LAMB2* and *WT1* genes are found in syndromic NS [27, 28, 29]. In a study with a large European cohort, 66% of the children presenting with NS in their first year of life were found to carry mutations in the *NPHS1*, *NPHS2*, *WT1* and *LAMB2* genes [30]. *WT1* mutations are associated with the Denys-Drash (DDS) and Frasier Syndromes (FS), whereas, mutations in the *LAMB2* gene cause Pierson syndrome [31]. Mutations in all the identified genes collectively account for a majority of the cases presenting with NS in their first year of life and also for childhood NS. Nonetheless, there is a sizeable minority of the cases whose genetic causes are still unknown. In spite of the identification of genes causing NS in children, there are certain loci that are reported to be associated with isolated NS as well as the syndromic forms of NS (Table 2).

NPHS1 Gene Mutations Associated with CNS and Early-onset NS

The *NPHS1* gene was first identified in 1998 by positional cloning method. It is located on chromosome 19q13.1 and contains 29 exons [27]. It encodes nephrin, which is a 185 KDa zipper-like transmembrane protein of the immunoglobin superfamily of cell adhesion molecules. It is characterized by eight C2-type Ig-like domains, a fibronectin type III repeat in the extracellular region, a single transmembrane domain and a cytosolic C-terminal end. It is expressed specifically in the podocytes where it's extracellular moiety forms homodimers and bridges the intercellular space between the podocyte foot processes forming the porous structure of the SD. Apart from its role as a structural component of the podocyte and the SD, it also plays an essential role in the intracellular signaling pathways where it interacts with certain other proteins like podocin, CD2 associated protein and TRPC6. Several other proteins have been reported to be associated with the nephrin- slit diaphragm complex to form a signaling platform around nephrin (Figure 3). It has been suggested that nephrin is critically involved in the signalling processes that are important for podocyte function, survival and differentiation [32].

The *NPHS1* gene was first identified as a cause of CNS in the Finnish population where two mutations, the Fin$_{major}$ (c.121deCT; p.L41fsX90) and the Fin$_{minor}$ (c.3325C>T; p.R1109X) account for 78% and 16% of the CNS cases respectively [27]. The CNS of the Finnish type (CNF) is characterized by a severe disease with onset in utero or within the first three months of life. It shows a typical renal histology with immature glomeruli, mesengial cell hypercellularity, pseudocystic dilations of the proximal tubules and foot process effacement. Most of the infants with CNF are born prematurely with low birth weight and an enlarged placenta. Edema is present at birth or appears within the first few days of life. Abnormal glomerular filtration can be detected prenatally as an increase in the maternal α-fetoproteins. Patients usually develop ESRD within 3-8 years. A number of children also die of complications of severe nephrosis (infection, thrombosis, intra-vascular volume depletion).

However, these two mutations are rarely found in other populations. *NPHS1* gene screening in non-Finnish populations has shown that the frequency of mutations is lower (~39 to 55%) in other populations compared to the Finnish patients. In total, more than 240 different mutations have been identified in the *NPHS1* gene in different populations of the world with variable frequencies [9, 30, 33–38]. These mutations include protein-truncating nonsense mutations, frameshift small insertion/deletion mutations and splice-site changes. Genotype-phenotype correlation studies have demonstrated a wide heterogeneity in the clinical course and severity of the disease phenotype associated with different mutations. Besides CNS, the *NPHS1* gene mutations have also been identified in patients with a milder disease of childhood onset with histological findings of FSGS [39, 40]. The clinical course can be explained by in vitro functional assays that have shown that most *NPHS1* missense mutations lead to the retention of protein in the endoplasmic reticulum due to the defective intracellular nephrin trafficking. This results in a complete loss of protein from the cell surface [41, 42]. In some cases, missense mutations with minor modifications that do not alter protein trafficking or dimerization, may produce a milder phenotype with onset of the disease later in life [39]. NS associated with the p.R1160X mutation show a severe as well as a milder phenotype that appears to be influenced by the gender of the patient as five out of the six patients reported were females [33]. Similarly, two siblings with severe CNS and compound heterozygous mutations in the *NPHS1* gene showed preserved renal function at the ages of 20 and 24 years [43]. It was initially thought that patients with a genetic cause of NS do not respond to drug therapy, but Patrakka et al.., (2000) reported their unique observation of significant decrease in proteinuria following the administration of angiotensin converting enzyme inhibitors and indomethacin in a girl with the Fin major mutation [44]. It is now evident that some patients may respond to the therapy and establish a partial or complete remission of proteinuria [38].

NPHS2 Gene Mutations Associated with CNS and Familial SRNS

The *NPHS2* gene was first mapped by classical linkage analysis in families with autosomal recessive SRNS to chromosome 1q25-q31 [45]. The coding region of the *NPHS2* gene is 1,149 bp in length and contains 8 exons. It codes for a 42-KDa protein podocin that localizes to the insertion site of the SD of podocytes. It consists of 383 amino acids with a cytosolic C– and an N– terminal domains and a short transmembrane domain. Podocin is an integral membrane protein of the stomatin family. It is highly expressed in the SD and is targeted to the plasma membrane where it forms homooligomers complexes. These complexes directly interact with cholesterol in specialized microdomains of the plasma membrane called lipid rafts. The association of podocin with these lipid raft microdomains is suggested to be a pre-requisite for the recruitment of nephrin into the lipid rafts [46].

Initially, the *NPHS2* gene was reported to cause familial early-onset NS with steroid-resistance and rapid progression to ESRD. Later, it is established that mutations in the podocin gene caused SRNS manifesting from birth to adulthood. Renal histology in most of the cases show FSGS, however, MCNS is also been identified in some cases. Phenotypes associated with the *NPHS2* mutations typically include early childhood onset of the disease, resistance to steroid treatment, progression to ESRD within 5 years of diagnosis, and a low risk of recurrence of the disease after transplantation [47, 48]. Studies with animal models show that *Nphs2* knockout mice are presented with a phenotype similar to human disease with foot process effacement, nephrotic range proteinuria and chronic renal insufficiency [49]. To date, more than 70 truncating, missense and splice site mutations have been reported in the *NPHS2* gene that cause NS. The *NPHS2* gene mutations are identified in 10 – 25% of the sporadic NS cases of childhood onset [47, 48]. The incidence in familial SRNS cases has been found to be 40% in the European and American children, 29% in the Turkish children and 0% in the Japanese, Korean and Pakistani children [38, 50]. Among the most frequent gene mutations, p.R138Q is typically associated with early-onset NS. The p.R138Q mutant podocin is shown to be retained in the endoplasmic reticulum and loses its ability to recruit nephrin in the lipid rafts [46]. Some other mutations (e.g., p.V180M and p.R238S) are found in patients with later onset SRNS suggesting that podocin may retain some function in these cases.

A frequently found single nucleotide polymorphism in the *NPHS2* gene is p.R229Q. It is shown to be present in varying frequencies in different populations of the world. It is found more frequently in the European populations (allele frequency from 2 to 7%) and less frequently in the populations of African descent from USA and Brazil (0.5 to 2.5% allele frequency). The allele frequencies in Asia and Africa are largely unknown. The pathogenic nature of this variant is extensively discussed in the literature. It is found in compound heterozygosity with another pathogenic mutation in the *NPHS2* gene in some cases of the SRNS/FSGS. These patients manifest NS later in life suggesting a reduced pathogenecity of this variant. The mutation was also found in a homozygous state in two children with childhood onset NS [38]. It is therefore considered to be a non-neutral variant that, when found with a second *NPHS2* mutation, tends to increase the chances of susceptibility to FSGS [51]. In vitro studies have demonstrated that the variant podocin shows a decreased binding capacity to the nephrin protein [51]. These observations emphasize the importance of this variant in the proper functioning of the protein. However, there are insufficient data to speculate that some gene variants like p.R229Q may also cause NS/FSGS.

A few studies also report a di-genic mode of inheritance where mutations in both the *NPHS1* and *NPHS2* genes are observed simultaneously [33, 38]. These observations provide the evidence of a functional relationship between the nephrin and podocin proteins and emphasize the critical role of these genes in maintaining the structural and functional integrity of the podocytes and GFB.

PLCE1 Gene Mutations Are Implicated in CNS and Recessive FSGS

The *PLCE1* gene spans 334 kb on chromosome 10 and contains 34 exons [52]. It encodes phospholipase C ε 1(PLC ε1), a member of phospholipase family of proteins that catalyzes the hydrolysis of phosphoinositides and generates second messengers such as IP3 and DAG. These second messengers regulate cell growth, differentiation and gene expression etc. [53]. The main function of IP3 is the stimulation of calcium release from intracellular storage pools. PLCE1 is involved in the cytoskeletal reorganization and is also shown to modulate the functions of other signal transduction cascade proteins. However, the precise mode of action of PLCE1 in the podocyte remains unclear.

The *PLCE1* gene mutations are the third most common cause of NS in infants after the *NPHS1* and *NPHS2* gene mutations [54]. Mutations in the *PLCE1* gene have been identified in 10 – 50% of the patients with NS and DMS and in 12% of the recessive familial FSGS cases [52, 55]. As the genetic forms of NS are thought to be non-responsive to steroid therapy, some patients carrying the *PLCE1* gene mutations show complete remission of proteinuria after the treatment with steroids and cyclosporine [52]. Hence, NS caused by *PLCE1* mutations may be regarded as drug-responsive NS. Another unique observation with *PLCE1* is the identification of homozygous mutations in asymptomatic individuals. A frameshift truncation mutation in exon 3 segregating in a family was also found in an asymptomatic adult. This phenomenon was explained by the presence of an unidentified genetic modifier that may compensate the PLCE1 defect [56].

WT1 Gene Causes Wilms' Tumor and Syndromic Forms of NS

The *WT1* gene is located on chromosome 11p13 and codes for a zinc-finger transcription factor important for the regulation of several genes involved in kidney and gonadal development [57, 58].

Mutations in the *WT1* gene have been known to cause Denys-Drash syndrome (DDS), Frasier syndrome (FS) and isolated NS with diffuse mesangial sclerosis (DMS) [59]. The DDS is characterized by the presence of early onset SRNS, XY pseudohermaphrodism, gonadal dysgenesis and Wilms' tumor (in more than 90% of the cases). The age of onset of SRNS is usually congenital. Patients rapidly progress to ESRD with a renal histology typical of DMS [60]. Electron microscopy shows foot process effacement. To prevent the development of Wilms' tumor, bilateral nephrectomy is usually recommended before the transplantation. No recurrence of disease has been observed after renal transplantation in the cases of *WT1* gene mutations [61]. Most of the mutations that are associated with the DDS phenotype are missense mutations, predominantly affecting exons 8 an9 of the *WT1* gene. Among these mutations, p.R394W is the most common mutation that affects the zinc finger domain and therefore reduces the DNA binding capacity of the WT1 protein. Knock-in mice with the heterozygous p.R394W mutation, have been shown to have DMS and male genital anomaly phenotypes that are characteristics of human DDS [62]. Isolated DMS has also been described to be associated with recessive *WT1* gene mutations [59].

The Frasier syndrome is also characterized by XY pseudohermaphrodism and progressive nephropathy with SRNS [63]. Patients with FS often show late onset proteinuria and a better renal outcome as compared to the patients with DDS. The patients present FSGS in renal biopsy and show good renal function until the second to third decade of life. They are presented with female external genitalia, streak gonads and XY karyotype [61]. The risk of developing Wilms' tumor is comparatively low in the patients with FS. However, the development of gonadoblastomata from gonadal dysgenesis is common. A heterozygous donor splice-site mutation in intron 9 has been associated with the FS phenotype. This mutation affects the KTS (lysine-threonine-serine amino acid residue) region of the WT1 protein and produces the KTS (–) isoform. The KTS (+) isoform of the WT1 protein has an important role in genitourinary and kidney development.

The truncating mutations in the *WT1* gene have been detected in the patients with isolated Wilms' tumor [64]. The Wilms' tumor is among the most common solid tumors in children and accounts for 8% of all the childhood cancers. The *WT1* gene mutations were first identified in the WAGR syndrome which is characterized by Wilms tumor, aniridia, genitourinary malformations and mental retardation (WAGR). Patients with the WAGR syndrome contain a deletion on the short arm of chromosome 11, associated with the complete loss of *WT1* function [65]. Familial type Wilms' tumor is also inherited in an autosomal dominant manner with germline mutations in the *WT1* gene. Patients carrying mutations show remarkable phenotypic heterogeneity. Splice site mutations that are found more frequently in the FS cases, are also identified in some cases of the DDS or in isolated DMS. Similarly, patients with mutations that are typical for DDS may exhibit isolated FSGS or Wilms' tumor [66, 67, 68]. Incomplete penetrance is also evident in some cases of the *WT1* gene mutations. Two monozygotic twins with a heterozygous p.R366P mutation died because of complications of CNS at 23 weeks and 13 months of age, respectively. Surprisingly, their father who was a carrier was asymptomatic and had normal renal function at the age of 41 years [69]. The possible explanation for this observation is described as the presence of somatic mosaicism or genomic imprinting or the lack of heritability [70, 71].

LAMB2 Gene Mutations Cause Pierson Syndrome As well As Isolated NS

The *LAMB2* gene codes for Laminin B2 protein that is crucial for podocyte foot process architecture and stability. It is widely expressed in the GBM, retina, lens capsule, intraocular muscle and the neuromuscular synapses. It is a laminin family member which are heterotrimeric glycoproteins consisting of α, β and γ subunits joined through a coiled coil [72]. They are essential components of all the basement membranes and play crucial roles in maintaining the structures of the basement membranes by forming a monolayer of laminins. They are also shown to mediate matrix-cell interactions that are involved in cell adhesion, differentiation and migration. The most important β2-containing laminin isoform is laminin-521 which is composed of α5, β2 and γ1 subunits and is specifically expressed in the GBM, intraocular muscles and neuromuscular synapses [73]. Laminin β 2 provides cross linking between the basolateral membranes of the podocyte to the GBM in the kidneys. Knock-out mice lacking the β2 chain exhibits proteinuria and die in the perinatal period [74]. Therefore, deficiency in the laminin β2 chain results in GBM alteration, functional impairment of the GFB and ocular anomalies.

Mutations in the *LAMB2* gene are associated with a rare autosomal recessive syndromic disorder, Pierson syndrome (OMIM #609049). It is characterized by the appearance of early onset NS and variable ocular and neurological defects. The typical ophthalmic signs in Pierson syndrome are microcoria (fixed narrowing of the pupils), abnormal lens shape with cataract and retinal abnormalities. Patients with severe phenotypes exhibit blindness and neuro-developmental defects including hypotonia and delayed motor and cognitive development [75]. Phenotypes of variable severity with less prominent ocular symptoms and isolated NS have also been described [76, 77]. The missense mutations and non-truncating deletion mutations in the *LAMB2* gene exhibit a relatively milder phenotype, while, patients with the protein truncating mutation show a severe phenotype with extrarenal manifestations.

Further, the patients with the mild phenotype show glomerulopathy with FSGS while, patients with the severe phenotype have diffuse mesengial sclerosis (DMS).

TRPC6 Gene Mutations Are Responsible to Cause Autosomal Dominant FSGS

The *TRPC6* gene is located on chromosome 11q21-q22. It encodes for the transient receptor cation channel TRPC6 and is expressed in podocytes, renal tubules and glomeruli. The TRPC6 protein consists of three or four amino-terminal ankyrin repeats, six putative transmembrane domains, a short sequence termed the "TRP box" (of unknown function), and a potential coiled-coil structures in the amino and carboxy sequences. The protein is thought to mediate the intracellular calcium homeostasis of the podocytes.

The mutant TRPC6 protein is implicated in impaired calcium signalling and shown to disrupt the glomerular cell function. It was first identified to cause autosomal dominant FSGS [78]. Mutations in the *TRPC6* gene account for 3-7% of the cases of familial adult-onset FSGS with mild to nephrotic range proteinuria, progressing to ESRD. Most of the mutations that have been reported so far are gain-of-function mutations leading to increased activity of ion channels by increasing the calcium current amplitudes or by delaying the channel inactivation. Recently *TRPC6* mutations have also been detected in patients with early to late onset SRNS with a unique association of collapsing glomerulosclerosis in renal histology in a 6 months old child [79].

ACTN4 Gene Mutations Cause Autosomal Dominant NS

The gene for α-actinin (*ACTN4*) is mapped to chromosome 19q3. It is an actin-bundling protein of the cytoskeleton and is highly expressed in the podocytes [80]. Initially, mutations in the *ACTN4* gene were identified in familial cases of autosomal dominant FSGS [81]. The affected family members were presented with adolescent onset proteinuria progressing to ESRD during adulthood. Renal histology revealed irregular granular staining patterns in the capillary walls of preserved glomeruli in patients with the *ACTN4* mutations. Incomplete penetrance is also observed in some members of these families without the development of renal phenotype suggesting the involvement of other genetic or non-genetic factors in the pathogenesis of *ACTN4* associated FSGS [81]. To date approximately ~150 gene mutations have been identified in the *ACTN4* gene (The 1000 genome browser, http://browser. 1000genomes.org/Homo_sapiens/Gene/Variation_Gene/) that are thought to interfere with the regulation of the actin cytoskeleton of podocytes. These mutations include missense and splice-site mutations frequently affecting the binding domain of actinin 4. However, mutations in the *ACTN4* gene account for only 4% of the familial cases of FSGS.

In vitro functional studies have demonstrated an increased binding of the mutant protein to the filamentous actin and the formation of large aggregates and impaired migration patterns [82, 83]. Recently it is shown that ACTN4 interacts with retinoic acid receptor (RARα) and enhances its transcriptional activation. In addition, mutant ACTN4 protein not only mislocalized to the cytoplasm, but it also loses its ability to be associated with nuclear receptors. Consequently, the mutant fails to potentiate transcriptional activation by the nuclear hormone receptors in podocytes [84].

INF2 Is Implicated in Autosomal Recessive FSGS and FSGS-associated Charcot-Marie-Tooth Disease (CMT)

A new locus for autosomal dominant FSGS was recently mapped on chromosome 14q containing the *INF2* gene by linkage analysis. INF2 is a member of the formin family of actin-regulating proteins that have been shown to accelerate the polymerization and depolymerization of actin in vitro [85]. It has an N-terminal diaphanous-inhibitory domain (DID), the forming homology domains FH1 and FH2, and a C-terminal diaphanous-autoregulatory domain (DAD).

The disease causing mutations identified in the *INF2* gene are missense mutations that are clustered in the DID and are shown to inhibit actin-depolymerization [86]. *INF2* mutations account for 9 - 16% of the cases of autosomal dominant familial FSGS. It was observed that INF2-related diseases showed variable penetrance with the onset of the disease ranging widely from childhood to adulthood and commonly leading to ESRD in the third and fourth decade of life [87, 88, 89]. Mutations in the *INF2* gene are also shown to be associated with the Charcot-Marie-Tooth disease (CMT). It is a group of inherited disorders affecting peripheral neurons and renal disease with FSGS [90].

Other Genes Causing Autosomal Recessive/Dominant NS/FSGS

Several other proteins have been identified to cause NS or associated glomerulopathies with and without extra renal manifestations and whose roles in the regulation of the GFB are less clear. Table 1 describes a list of genes that are known to be associated with NS and FSGS. The *CD2AP* gene codes for an actin-related protein and in homozygous knock-out mice mutations in this gene are shown to cause DMS and renal failure. Subsequently, autosomal dominant mutations in the *CD2AP* were identified to cause FSGS [91]. Mutations have been identified in the *PTPRO* gene in a study of SRNS families of Turkish and non-Turkish origins [92]. Notably, children with the homozygous *PTPRO* gene mutations are responsive to intensified immunosuppressive treatment. PTPRO is a tyrosine phosphatase and is expressed at the apical membrane of the podocyte foot processes. Tyrosine phosphorylation of tight junction proteins are shown to play a major role in controlling the paracellular permeability, cell signaling, and actin cytoskeleton remodeling [92]. Mutations in the *MYO1E* gene have been identified to be associated with childhood-onset, glucocorticoid-resistant FSGS [93]. Electron microscopy of children with the *MYO1E* mutations showed thickening and disorganization of the glomerular basement membrane.

Renal Transplantation and Genetic Counseling

The patients with SRNS usually develop ESRD and require dialysis and/or renal transplantation. It is estimated that about 30% of the pediatric SRNS patients with a renal histology of FSGS show recurrence of the disease after transplantation [94, 95]. The recurrence of proteinuria is seen as early as 14 day post transplantation. Higher recurrence rate is shown in children when the age of disease onset is more than 6 years. However, in these patients treatments with cyclophosphamide and plasmapheresis have been shown to be useful. In the cases of *NPHS1* gene mutations, the recurrence of proteinuria is shown to be due to the development of antibodies to nephrin in the recipients [96, 97]. It is also suggested that a T-cell derived circulating plasma factor may be responsible for the recurrence of proteinuria [98]. Another factor called serum glomerular permeability factor is also observed as a cause of recurrent proteinuria [99]. However, the recurrence of the disease following renal transplantation is less frequent (10%) in the hereditary NS cases with the clinical presentation of FSGS. Among these, patients with *NPHS1* gene mutations have a comparatively higher risk of recurrence which is equal to those with idiopathic FSGS, whereas patients with the *NPHS2* gene mutation show a low rate of recurrence.

Living-related donor transplantation is often considered as the therapy of first choice in pediatric SRNS patients. However, due to the scarcity of data regarding the outcome of transplant in hereditary SRNS, there is a need to evaluate large cohorts of patients for the function and performance of the donor organs in the recipients and the remaining single kidney in the donors. Currently, the significance of single heterozygous mutation in most of the NS cases is unknown, and the susceptibility to develop the disease in these patients is unclear. Therefore, the kidney from a carrier parent may cause susceptibility for the disease and also the living donor with one kidney may be at risk for NS/FSGS. Genetic testing for the other family members should be done in order to identify the carriers before transplantation. In the case of the dominant disorder, only one parent carries the mutation, the other parent with the two normal alleles can be regarded as a suitable donor. Genetic counseling should be offered to the families segregating SRNS/FSGS because of the risk of recurrence of the disease (25% in recessive and 50% in dominant disease). It is also recommended because in contrast to sporadic NS, patients with hereditary NS show a more severe phenotype with resistance to corticosteroid therapy and rapid progression to ESRD. Genotype-phenotype correlation studies, therefore, prove to be helpful in facilitating genetic counseling and establishing the clinical course in other affected members of the family.

The most important aspect of such genetic studies is the use of this information in understanding the physiology of the podocytes and GFB as well as the pathophysiology of nephrotic syndrome. There is a need to find the genetic causes of the remaining cases of NS and the pathways that are altered in the etiology of the disease. Currently employed new technologies such as whole genome sequencing (WGS), next generation sequencing (NGS) will allow the rapid and comprehensive screening of the genes and loci that remain unidentified. Collaborative research work is probably the key to the success in the identification of genetic causes and the exploration of the etiologies of the disease. Several collaborative research consortia and study groups are working together to find curative strategies for NS, the adverse effects of drug therapies and to provide high quality health care. These groups includes, the Study Group of the Arbeitsgemeinschaft fur Padiatrische

Nephrologie (APN), the PodoNet Consortium (http://www.podonet.org), the Nephcure Foundation (http://www.nephcure.org), the nephrotic syndrome registry (http://www.nsregistry.org) and the North American initiatives (Neptune, http://rarediseases network.epi.usf.edu/NEPTUNE) etc. These registries and research groups are involved in integrated research to obtain genotypic and phenotypic information from geographically and ethnically different cohorts of patients.

Acknowledgment

I would like to thank Professor Syed Qasim Mehdi for his support and critical reading of the manuscript.

Conflict of Interests

The author declares no conflict of interest.

References

[1]   Jarad G and Miner JH: Update on the glomerular filtration barrier. *Curr Opin Nephrol Hypertens. 18*, 226-232 (2009).

[2]   Zenker M, Machuca E and Antignac C: Genetics of nephrotic syndrome: new insights into molecules acting at the glomerular filtration barrier. *J Mol Med. 87*, 849-857 (2009).

[3]   Yu Z, Ding J, Huang J, Yao Y, Xiao H, Zhang J, Liu J and Yang J: Mutations in NPHS2 in sporadic steroid resistant nephrotic syndrome in Chinese children. *Nephrol Dial Transplant 20(5)*, 902-908 (2005).

[4]   Gipson DS, Chin H, Presler TP, Jennette C, Ferris ME, Massengill S, Gibson K, Thomas DB. Differential risk of remission and ESRD in childhood FSGS. *Pediatr Nephrol. 21*, 344-349 (2006).

[5]   Greenbaum LA, Benndorf R and Smoyer WE. Childhood nephrotic syndrome-current and future therapies. *Nat Rev Nephrol. 8*, 445-458 (2012).

[6]   Buscher AK, Kranz B, Büscher R, Hildebrandt F, Dworniczak B, Pennekamp P, Kuwertz-Bröking E, Wingen AM, John U, Kemper M, Monnens L, Hoyer PF, Weber S, Konrad M. Immunosuppression and renal outcome in congenital and pediatric steroid-resistant nephrotic syndrome. *Clin J Am Soc Nephrol. 5(11)*, 2075-2084 (2010).

[7]   Eddy AA, Symons JM. Nephrotic syndrome in childhood. *Lancet. 362(9384)*, 629-639 (2003).

[8]   Bolk S, Puffenberger EG, Hudson J, Morton DH, Chakravarti A. Elevated frequency and allelic heterogeneity of congenital nephrotic syndrome, Finnish type, in the old order Mennonites. *Am J Hum Genet. 65(6)*, 1785-1790 (1999).

[9]   Beltcheva O, Martin P, Lenkkeri U, Tryggvason K. Mutation spectrum in the nephrin gene (NPHS1) in congenital nephrotic syndrome. *Hum Mutat. 17(5),* 368-373 (2001).

[10] Wong W. Idiopathic nephrotic syndrome in New Zealand children demographic, clinical features, initial management and outcome after twelve-month follow-up: results of a three year national survelliance study. *J Paediatr Child Health. 43(5),* 337-341 (2007).

[11] Ingulli E, Tejani A. Racial differences in the incidence and renal outcome of idiopathic focal segmental glomerulosclerosis in children. *Pediatr Nephrol. 5(4),* 393-397 (1991).

[12] Boyer O, Moulder JK, Somer MJ. Focal and segmental glomerulosclerosis in children: a longitudinal assessment. *Pediatr Nephrol. 22(8),* 1159-1166 (2007).

[13] Sharples PM, Poulton J, White RH. Steroid responsive NS is more common in Asians. *Arch Dis Child. 60,* 1014-1017 (1985).

[14] Coovadia HM, Adhikari M, Morel-Maroger L. Clinico-pathological features of the nephrotic syndrome in South African children. *Quarterly Journal of Medicine. 48(189),* 77-91 (1979).

[15] Abdurrahman MB, Aikhionbare HA, Babaoye FA, Sathiakumar N, Narayana PT. Clinicopathological features of childhood nephrotic syndrome in Northern Nigeria. *Quarterly Journal of Medicine. 75(278),* 563-576 (1990).

[16] Niaudet P. Steroid-sensitive idiopathic nephrotic syndrome in children. In: Avner E, Harmon W and Niaudet P. Pediatric Nephrology. 5th ed. Philadelphia: Lippincott, Williams and Wilkins; 2004

[17] Filler G, Young E, Geier P, Carpenter B, Drukker A, Feber J. Is there really an increase in non-minimal change nephrotic syndrome in children? *A J Kidney Disease. 42(6),* 1107-1113 (2003).

[18] International Study of Kidney Diseases in Children: Nephrotic syndrome in children: prediction of histopathology from clinical and laboratory characteristics at time of diagnosis, *Kidney Int. 13,* 159-165 (1978).

[19] Borges FF Shiraichi L, da Silva MP, Nishimoto EI, Nogueira PCK. Is focal segmental glomerulosclerosis increasing in patients with nephrotic syndrome? *Pediatr Nephrol. 22,* 1309-1313 (2007).

[20] The primary nephrotic syndrome in children: identification of patients with minimal change nephrotic syndrome from initial response to prednisone. A report of the International Study of Kidney Disease in children. *J Pediatr. 98,* 561-564 (1981a).

[21] Kumar J, Gulati S, Sharma AP, Sharma RK, Gupta RK. Histopathological spectrum of childhood nephrotic syndrome in Indian children. *Pediatr Nephrol. 18,* 657-660 (2003).

[22] Mubarak M, Lanewala A, Kazi JI, Akhter F, Sher A, Fayyaz A and Bhatti Sajid: Histological spectrum of childhood nephrotic syndrome in Pakistan. *Clinical Exp Nephrol. 13(6),* 589-593 (2009).

[23] The primary nephrotic syndrome in children: clinical significance of histopathologic variants of minimal change and of diffuse mesengial hypercellularity. A report of the International Study of Kidney Disease in children. *Kidney Int. 20,* 765-771 (1981b).

[24] Avni EF, Vandenhoute K, Devriendt A, Ismaili K, Hackx M, Janssen F and hall M: Update on congenital nephrotic syndromes and the contribution of US. *Pediatr Radiol. 41,* 76-81 (2011).

[25] Goldenberg A, Ngoc LH, Thouret MC, Cormier-Daire V, Gagnadoux MF, Chretien D, Lefrancois C, Geromel V, Rotig A, Rustin P, Munnich A, Paquis V, Antignac C,

Gubler MC, Niaudet P, Lonlay P. Berard E. Respiratory chain deficiency presenting as congenital nephrotic syndrome. *Pediatr Nephrol. 20*, 465-469 (2005).

[26] Buscher AK and Weber S. Educational paper: The podocytopathies. *Eur J Pediatr. 171(8)*, 1151-1160 (2012).

[27] Kestila M, Lenkkeri U, Mannikko M, Lamerdin J, McCready P, Putaala H, Ruotsalainen V, Morita T, Nissinen M, Herva R, Kashtan CE, Peltonen L, Holmberg C, Olsen A, Tryggvason K. Positionally cloned gene for a novel glomerular protein-nephrin-is mutated in congenital nephrotic syndrome. *Mol Cell. 1(4)*, 575-582 (1998).

[28] Boute N, Gribouval O, Roselli S, Benessy F, Lee H, Fuschshuber A, dahan K, Gubler MC, Niaudet P, Antignac C. NPHS2 encoding the glomerular protein, podocin, is mutated in autosomal recessive steroid-resistant nephrotic syndrome. *Nat Genet. 24*, 349-354 (2000).

[29] Machuca E, Benoit G, Antignac C. Genetics of nephrotic syndrome: connecting molecular genetics to podocyte physiology. *Hum Mol Genet. 18*, 185-194 (2009).

[30] Hinkes BG, Mucha B, Vlangos CN, Gbadegesin R, Liu J, Hesselbacher K, Hangan D, Ozaltin F, Zenker M, Hildebrandt F. Nephrotic syndrome in the first year of life: two thirds of cases are caused by mutations in 4 genes (NPHS1, NPHS2, WT1 and LAMB2). *Pediatrics. 119*, e907-e919 (2007).

[31] Barbaux S, Niaudet P, Gubler MC, Grunfeld JP, Jaubert F, Kuttenn F, Fekete CN, Souleyreau-Therville N, Thibaud E, Fellous M, McElreavey K. Donor splice-site mutations in WT1 are responsible for Frasier syndrome. *Nat Genet. 17*, 467-470 (1997).

[32] Patrakka J, Tryggvason K. Nephrin- a unique structural and signaling protein of the kidney filter. *Trends Mol Med. 13*, 396-403 (2007).

[33] Koziell A, Grech V, Hussain S, Lee G, Lenkkeri U. Tryggvason K and Scambler P: Genotype/phenotype correlations of *NPHS1* and *NPHS2* mutations in nephrotic syndrome advocate a functional inter-relationship in glomerular filtration. *Hum Mol Genet. 11(4)*, 379-388 (2002).

[34] Sako M, Nakanishi K, Obana M, Yata N, Hoshii S, Takahashi S, Wada N, Takahashi Y, Kaku Y, Satomura K, Ikeda M, Honda M, Iijima K, Yoshikawa N. Analysis of NPHS1, NPHS2, ACTN4 and WT1 in Japanese patients with congenital nephrotic syndrome. *Kidney Int. 67*, 1248-1255 (2005).

[35] Heeringa SF, Vlangos CN, Chernin G, Hinkes B, Gbadegesin R, Liu J, Hoskins BE, Ozaltin F, Hildebrandt F. Thirteen novel NPHS1 mutations in a large cohort of children with congenital nephrotic syndrome. *Nephrol Dial Transplant. 23*, 3527-3533 (2008).

[36] Ismaili K, Pawtowski A, Boyer O, Wissing KM, Janssen F, Hall M. Genetic forms of nephrotic syndrome: a single-center experience in Brussels. *Pediatr Nephrol. 24*, 287-294 (2009).

[37] Machuca E, Benoit G, Nevo F, Tete MJ, Gribouval O, Pawtowski A, Brandstrom P, Loirat C, Niaudet P, Gubler MC, Antignac C. Genotype phenotype correlations in non-Finnish congenital nephrotic syndrome. *J Am Soc Nephrol. 21*, 1209-1217 (2010).

[38] Abid A, Khaliq S, Shahid S, Lanewala A, Mubarak M, Hashmi S, Kazi J, Masood T, Hafeez F, Naqvi SAA, Rizvi SA, Mehdi SQ. A spectrum of novel *NPHS1* and *NPHS2* gene mutations in pediatric nephrotic syndrome patients from Pakistan. *Gene. 502(2)*, 133-137 (2012).

[39] Philippe A, Nevo F, Esquivel EL, Reklaityte D, Gribouval O, Tete MJ, Loirat C, Dantal J, Fischbach M, Pouteil-Noble C, Decramer S, Hoehne M, Benzing T, Charbit M, Niaudet P, Antignac C. Nephrin mutations can cause childhood onset steroid-resistant nephrotic syndrome. *J Am Soc Nephrol. 19(10)*, 1871-1878 (2008).

[40] Santin S, Garcia-Maset R, Ruiz P, Gimenez I, Zamora I, Pena A, Madrid A, Camacho JA, Fraga G, Sanchez-Moreno A, Cobo MA, Bernis C, Ortiz A, de Pablos AL, Pintos G, Justa ML, Hidalgo-Barquero E, Fernandez-Llama P, Ballarin J, Ars E, Torra R; FSGS Spanish Study Group. Nephrin mutations cause childhood and adult-onset focal segmental glomerulosclerosis. *Kidney Int. 76(12)*, 1268-1276 (2009).

[41] Liu XL, Done SC, Khoshnoodi J, Bertorello A, Wartiovaara J, Berggren PO, Tryggvason K. Defective nephrin trafficking caused by missense mutations in the NPHS1 gene: insights into the mechanisms of congenital nephrotic syndrome. *Hum Mol Genet. 10*, 2637-2644 (2001).

[42] Liu XL, Done SC, Yan K, Kilpelainen P, pikkarainen T, Tryggvason K. Defective trafficking of nephrin missense mutants rescue by a chemical chaperone. *J Am Soc Nephrol. 15*, 1731-1738 (2004).

[43] Schulteisss M, Ruf RG, Mucha BE, Wiggins R, Fuchshuber A, Lichtenberger A, Hildebrandt F. No evidence for genotype/phenotype correlation in NPHS1 and NPHS2 mutations. *Padiatr Nephrol. 19(12)*, 1340-1348 (2004).

[44] Patrakka J, Kestila M, Wartiovaara J, Ruotsalainen V, Tissari P, Lenkkeri U, Mannikko M, Visapaa I, Holmberg C, Rapola J, Tryggvason K, Jalanko H. Congenital nephrotic syndrome (NPHS1); features resulting from different mutations in Finnish patients. *Kidney Int. 58*, 972-980 (2000).

[45] Fuchshuber A, Jean G, Gribouval O, Gubler MC, Broyer M, Beckmann JS, Niaudet P, Antignac C. Mapping of a gene (SRN1) to chromosome 1q25-q31 in idiopathic nephrotic syndrome confirms a distinct entity of autosomal recessive nephrosis. *Hum Mol Genet. 4(11)*, 2155-2158 (1995).

[46] Huber TB, Simons M, hartleben B, Semetz L, Schmidts M, Gundlach E, Saleem MA, Walz G and Benzing T. Molecular basis of the functional podocin-nephrin complex: mutations in the *NPHS2* gene disrupt nephrin targeting to lipid raft microdomains. *Hum Mol Genet. 12(24)*, 3397-3405 (2003).

[47] Ruf RG, Lichtenberger A, Karle SM, Haas JP, Anacleto FE, Schultheiss M, Zalewski I, Imm A, Ruf EM, Mucha B, Bagga A, Neuhaus T, Fuchshuber A, Bakkaloglu A, Hildebrandt F; Arbeitsgemeinschaft Für Pädiatrische Nephrologie Study Group. Patients with mutations in NPHS2 (podocin) do not respond to standard steroid treatment of nephrotic syndrome. *J Am Soc Nephrol. 15(3)*, 722-732 (2004).

[48] Weber S Gribouval O, Esquivel EL, Morinière V, Tête MJ, Legendre C, Niaudet P, Antignac C. NPHS2 mutation analysis shows genetic heterogeneity of steroid resistant nephrotic syndrome and low post-transplant recurrence. *Kidney Int. 66(2)*, 571-579 (2004).

[49] Roselli S, Heidet L, Sich M, Henger A, Kretzler M, Gubler MC, Antignac C. Early glomerular filtration defect and severe renal disease in podocin-deficient mice. *Mol Cell Biol. 24(2)*, 550-560 (2004).

[50] Lowik MM, Groenen PJ, Levtchenko EN, Monnens LA and van den Heuvel LP: Molecular genetic analysis of podocyte genes in focal segmental glomerulosclerosis. *Eur J Pediatr. 168*, 1291-1304 (2009).

[51] Tsukaguchi H, Sudhakar A, Le TC, Nguyen T, Yao J, Schwimmer JA, Schachter AD, Poch E, Abreu PF, Appel GB, Pereira AB, Kelluri R, Pollak MR. NPHS2 mutations in late-onset focal segmental glomerulosclerosis: R229Q is a common disease associated allele. *J Clin Invest. 110(11)*, 1659-1666 (2002).

[52] Hinkes B, Wiggins RC, Gbadegesin R, Vlangos CN, Seelow D, Nurnberg G, Garg P, Verma R, Chaib H, Hoskins BE, Ashraf S, Becker C, Hennies HC, Goyal M, Wharram BL, Schachter AD, Mudumana S, Drummond I, Kerjaschki D, Waldherr R, Dietrich A, Ozaltin F, Bakkaloglu A, Cleper R, Basel-Vanagaite L, pohl M, Griebel M, Tsygin AN, Soylu A, Muller D, Sorli CS, Bunney TD, Katan M, Liu J, Attanasio M, O'Toole JF, Hasselbacher K, Mucha B, Otto EA, Airik R, Kispert A, Kelley GG, Smrcka AV, Gudermann T, Holzman LB, Nurnberg P, Hildebrandt F. Positional cloning uncovers mutations in PLCE1 responsible for a nephrotic syndrome variant that may be reversible. *Nat Genet. 38*, 1397-1405 (2006).

[53] Hinkes BG. NPHS3: New clues for understanding idiopathic nephrotic syndrome. *Pediatr Nephrol. 23,* 847-850 (2008).

[54] Gbadegesin R, Hinkes BG, Hoskins BE, Vlangos CN, Heeringa SF Liu J, Loirat C, Ozaltin F, Hashmi S, Ulmer F, Cleper R, Ettenger R, Antignac C, Wiggins RC, Zenker M, Hildebrandt F. Mutations in PLCE1 are a major cause of isolated diffuse mesangial sclerosis (IDMS). *Nephrol Dial Transplant. 23*, 1291-1297 (2008).

[55] Boyer O, Benoit G, Gribouval O, Nevo F, Pawtowski A, Bilge I, Bircan Z, Deschenes G, Guay-Woodford LM, Hall M, Macher MA, Soulami K, Stefanidis CJ, Weiss R, Loirat C, Gubler MC, Antignac C. Mutational analysis of the PLCE1 gene in steroid resistant nephrotic syndrome. *J Med Genet. 47*, 445-452 (2012).

[56] Gilbert RD, Turner CL., Gibson J, Bass PS, Haq MR, Cross E, Bunyan DJ, Collins AR, Tapper WJ, Needell JC, Dell B, Morton NE, Temple IK, Robinson DO. Mutations in phospholipase C epsilon 1 are not sufficient to cause diffuse mesangial sclerosis. *Kidney Int. 75*, 415-419 (2009).

[57] Call KM, Glaser T, Ito CY, Buckler AL, Pelletier J, Haber DA, Rose EZ, Kari A, Yeger H, lewis WH, Jones C, Housman DE. Isolation and characterization of zinc finger polypeptide gene at the human chromosome 11 Wilms' tumor locus. *Cell. 60*, 509-520 (1990).

[58] Rose EA, Glaser T, Jones C, Smith CL, Lewis WH, Call KM, Minden M, Champagne E, Bonetta L, Yeger H, Housman DE. Complete physical map of the WAGR region of 11p13 localizes a candidate Wilms' tumor gene. *Cell. 60(3)*, 495-508 (1990).

[59] Jeanpierre C, Denamur E, Henry I, Cabanis MO, Luce S, Cecille A, Elion J, Peuchmaur M, Loirat C, Niaudet P, Gubler MC, Junien C. Identification of constitutional WT1 mutations, in patients with isolated diffuse mesangial sclerosis, and analysis of genotype/phenotype correlations by use of a computerized mutation database. *Am J Hum Genet. 62(4)*, 824-833 (1998).

[60] Habib R, Gubler MC, Antignac C, Gagnadoux MF. Diffuse mesangial sclerosis: a congenital glomerulopathy with nephrotic syndrome. *Adv Nephrol Necker Hosp. 22*, 43-57 (1993).

[61] Niaudet P, Gubler MC. *WT1* and gromerular disease. *Pediatr Nephrol. 21*, 1653-1660 (2006).

[62] Gao F, Maiti S, Sun G, Ordonez NG, Udtha M, Deng JM, Behringer RR, Huff V. The WT1 +/R394W mouse displays glomerulosclerosis and early-onset renal failure

characteristic of human Denys-Drash syndrome. *Mol Cell Biol. 24(22)*, 9899-9910 (2004).

[63] Moorthy AV, Chesney RW, Lubinsky M. Chronic renal failure and XY gonadal dysgenesis: "Frasier" syndrome – a commentary on reported cases. *Am J Med Genet. 3*, 297-302 (1987).

[64] Haber DA, Buckler AJ, Glaser T, Call KM, Pelletier J, Sohn RL, Douglass EC, Housmann DE. An internal deletion within an 11p13 zinc finger gene contributes to the development of Wilm's tumor. *Cell. 61(7)*, 1257-1269 (1990).

[65] Gessler M, Burns GA. Molecular mapping and cloning of the breakpoints of a chromosome 11p14.1-p13 deletion associated with the AGR syndrome. *Genomics. 3(2)*, 117-122 (1988).

[66] Pelletier J, Bruening W, Kashtan CE, Mauer SM, Manivel JC, Striegel JE, Houghton DC, Junien C, Habib R, Fouser L, Fine RN, Silverman BL, Haber DA, Housman D. Germline mutations in the Wilms' tumor suppressor gene are associated with abnormal urogenital development in Denys-Drash syndrome. *Cell. 67(2)*, 437-447 (1991).

[67] Kaplinsky C, Ghahremani M, Frishberg Y, Rechavi G, Pelletier J. Familial Wilms' tumor associated with a WT1 zinc finger mutation. *Genomics. 38(3)*, 451-453 (1996).

[68] Denamur E, Bocquet N, Baudouin V, Da Silva F, Veitia R, Peuchmaur M, Elion J, Gubler MC, Fellous M, Niaudet P, Loirat C. WT1 splice-site mutations are rarely associated with primary steroid resistant focal and segmental glomerulosclerosis. *Kidney Int. 57(5)*, 1868-1872 (2000).

[69] Fencl F, malina M, stara V, Zieg J, Mixova D, Seeman T, Blahova K. Discordant expression of a new WT1 gene mutation in a family with monozygotic twins presenting with congenital nephrotic syndrome. *Eur J Pediatr. 171(1)*, 121-124 (2012).

[70] Coppes MJ, Liefers GJ, Higuchi M, Zinn AB, Balfe JW, Williams BR. Inherited WT1 mutation in Denys-Drash syndrome. *Cancer Res. 52(21)*, 6125-6128 (1992).

[71] Little SE, Hanks SP, King-Underwood L, Jones C, Rapley EA, Rahman N, Pritchard-Jones K. Frequency and heritability of WT1 mutations in nonsyndromic Wilms' tumor patients: a UK Children's Cancer Study Group Study. *J Clin Oncol. 22(20)*, 4140-4146 (2004).

[72] Tunggal P, Smyth N, Paulsson M, Ott MC. Laminins: structure and genetic regulation. *Microsc Res Tech. 51*, 214-227 (2000).

[73] Miner JH, Patton BL. Laminin 11. *Int J Biochem Cell Biol. 31*, 811-816 (1999).

[74] Noakes PG, Miner JH, Gautam M, Cunningham JM, Sanes JR, Merlie JP. The renal glomerulus of mice lacking s-laminin/Laminin β2: nephrosis despite molecular compensation by lamini β1. *Nat Genet. 10*, 400-406 (1995).

[75] Wuhl E, Kogan J, Zurowska A, Matejas V, Vandevoorde RG, Aigner T, Wendler O, Lesniewska I, Bouvier R, Reis A, Weis J, Cochat P, Zenker M. Neurodevelopmental deficits in Pierson (microcoria-congenital nephrosis) syndrome. *Am J Med Genet A. 143*, 311-319 (2007).

[76] Choi HJ, Lee BH, Kang JH, Jeong HJ, Moon KC, Ha IS, Yu YS, Matejas V, Zenker M, Choi Y, Cheong HI. Variable phenotype of Pierson syndrome. *Pediatr Nephrol. 23*, 995-1000 (2008).

[77] Matejas V, Hinkes B, Alkandari F, Al-Gazali L, Annexstad E, Aytac MB, Barrow m, Blahova K, Bockenhauer D, Cheong HI, Maruniak-Chudek I, Cochat P, Dotsch J, Gajjar P, Hennekam RC, Janssen F, Kagan M, Kariminejad A, Kemper MJ, Koenig J, Kogan

J, Kroes HY, Kuwertz-Broking E, Lewanda AF, Medeira A, Muscheites J, Niaudet P, Pierson M, Saggar A, Seaver L, Suri M, Tsygin A, Wuhl E, Zurowska A, Uebe S, Hildebrandt F, Antignac C, Zenker M. Mutations in the human Laminin B2 (LAMB2) gene and the associated phenotypic spectrum. *Human Mutation. 31(9)*, 992-1002 (2010).

[78] Winn MP, Conlon PJ, Lynn KL, Farrington MK, Creazzo T, Hawkins AF, daskalakis N, Kwan SY, Ebersviller S, Burchette JL, Pericak-Vance MA, Howell DN, Vance JM, Rosenberg PB. Amutation in the TRPC6 cation channel causes familial focal segmental glomerulosclerosis. *Science. 308*, 1801-1804 (2005).

[79] Gigante M, Caridi G, Montemurno E, Soccio M, D'Apolito m, Cerullo G, Aucella F, Schirinzi A, Emma F, Massella L, Messina G, de Palo T, ranieri E, Ghiggeri GM, Gesulado L. TRPC6 mutations in children with steroid resistant nephrotic syndrome and atypical phenotype. *Clin J Am Soc Nephrol. 6(7)*, 1626-1634 (2011).

[80] Mathis BJ, Kim SH, Calabrese K, Haas M, Seidman JG, Seidman CE, pollak MR. A locus for inherited focal segmental glomerulosclerosis maps to chromosome 19q13. *Kidney Int. 53(2)*, 282-286 (1998).

[81] Kaplan JM, Kim SH, North KN, Rennke H, Correia LA, Tong HQ, Mathis BJ, Rodriguez-Perez JC, Allen PG, Beggs AH, Pollak MR. Mutations in ACTN4, encoding alpha-actinin-4, cause familial focal segmental glomerulosclerosis. *Nat Genet. 24(3)*, 251-256 (2000).

[82] Yao J, Le TC, Kos CH, Henderson JM, Allen PG, Denker BM, Pollak MR. Alpha-actinin-4-mediated FSGS: an inherited kidney disease caused by an aggregated and rapidly degraded cytoskeletal protein. *PLoS Biol. 2(6)*, e167 (2004).

[83] Michaud JL, Chaisson KM, Parks RJ, Kennedy CR. FSGS-associated alpha-actinin-4 (K256E) impairs cytoskeletal dynamics in podocytes. *Kidney Int. 70(6)*, 1054-1061 (2006).

[84] Khurana S, Chakraborty S, Lam M, Liu Y, Su YT, Zhao X, Saleem MA, Mathieson PW, Bruggeman LA, Kao HY. Familial focal segmental glomerulosclerosis (FSGS)-linked α-actinin 4 (ACTN4) protein mutants lose ability to activate transcription by nuclear hormone receptors. *J Biol Chem. 287(15)*, 12027-12035 (2012).

[85] Higgs HN. Formin proteins: a domain-based approach. *Trends Biochem Sci. 30(6)*, 342-353 (2005).

[86] Chhabra ES, Ramabhadran V, Gerber SA, Higgs HN. INF2 is an endoplasmic reticulum-soociated formin protein. *J Cell Sci. 122(9)*, 1430-1440 (2009).

[87] Brown EJ, Schlondorff JS, Becker DJ, Tsukaguchi H, Tonna SJ, Uscinski AL, Higgs HN, Henderson JM, Pollak MR. Mutation in the formin gene INF2 cause focal segmental glomerulosclerosis. *Nat Genet. 42*, 72-76 (2010).

[88] Barura M, Brown EJ, Charoonratana VT, Genovese G, Sun H, Pollak MR, Mutations in the INF2 gene account for a significant proportion of familial but not sporadic focal and segmental glomerulosclerosis. *Kidney Int.* 2012; *doi: 10.1038/ki.2012.349.* [Epub ahead of print]

[89] Gbadegesin R, , Lavin PJ, Hall G, Bartkowiak B, Homstad A, Jiang R, Wu G, Byrd A, Lynn K, Wolfish N, Ottati C, Stevens P, Howell D, Conlon P, Winn MP. Inverted formin 2 mutations with variable expression in patients with sporadic and hereditary focal and segmental glomerulosclerosis. *Kidney Int. 81(1)*, 94-99 (2012).

[90] Boyer O, Nevo F, Plaisier E, Funalot B, Gribouval O, Benoit G, Cong EH, Arrondel C, Tête MJ, Montjean R, Richard L, Karras A, Pouteil-Noble C, Balafrej L, Bonnardeaux A, Canaud G, Charasse C, Dantal J, Deschenes G, Deteix P, Dubourg O, Petiot P, Pouthier D, Leguern E, Guiochon-Mantel A, Broutin I, Gubler MC, Saunier S, Ronco P, Vallat JM, Alonso MA, Antignac C, Mollet G. INF2 mutations in Charcot-Marie-Tooth disease with glomerulopathy. *New Eng J Med. 365(25)*, 2377-2388 (2011).

[91] Gigante M, Pontrelli P, Montemurno E, Roca L, Aucella F, Penza R, Caridi G, Ranieri E, Ghiggeri GM, Gesualdo L. CD2AP mutations are associated with sporadic nephrotic syndrome and focal segmental glomerulosclerosis (FSGS). *Nephrol Dial Transplant. 24*, 1858-1864 (2009).

[92] Ozaltin F, Ibsirlioglu T, Taskiran EZ, Baydar DE, Kaymaz F, Buyukcelik M, Kilic BD, Balat A, Iatropoulos P, Asan E, Akarsu NA, Schaefer F, Yilmaz E, Bakkaloglu A; PodoNet Consortium. Disruption of PTPRO causes childhood onset nephrotic syndrome. *Am J Hum Genet. 89*, 139-147 (2011).

[93] Mele C, Mele C, Iatropoulos P, Donadelli R, Calabria A, Maranta R, Cassis P, Buelli S, Tomasoni S, Piras R, Krendel M, Bettoni S, Morigi M, Delledonne M, Pecoraro C, Abbate I, Capobianchi MR, Hildebrandt F, Otto E, Schaefer F, Macciardi F, Ozaltin F, Emre S, Ibsirlioglu T, Benigni A, Remuzzi G, Noris M; PodoNet Consortium. *MYO1E* Mutations and Childhood Familial Focal Segmental Glomerulosclerosis. *New Eng J Med. 365(4)*, 295-306 (2011).

[94] Artero M, Biava C, Amend W, Tomlanovich S, Vincenti F. Recurrent focal segmental glomerulosclerosis: natural history and response to therapy, *Am J Med. 92(4)*, 375-383 (1992).

[95] Cochat P, fargue S, mestrallet G, jungraithmayr T, Koch-Nogueira P, Ranchin B, Zimmerhackl LB. disease recurrence in pediatric renal transplantation. *Pediatr Nephrol. 24*, 2097-2108 (2009).

[96] Wang SX, Ahola H, Palmen T Solin ML, Luimula P, Holthöfer H Recurrence of nephrotic syndrome after transplantation in CNF is due to autoantibodies to nephrin. *Exp Nephrol. 9*, 327-331 (2001).

[97] Patrakka J, Ruotsalainen V, Reponen P, Qvist E, laine J, Holmberg C, Tryggvason K, Jalanko H. Recurrence of nephrotic syndrome in kidney grafts of patients with congenital nephrotic syndrome of the Finnish type: role of nephrin. *Transplantation. 73*, 394-403 (2002).

[98] Savin VJ, Sharma R, Sharma M, McCarthy ET, Swan SK, Ellis E, Lovell H, Warady B, Gunwar S, Chonko AM, Artero M, Vincenti F. Circulating factor associated with increased glomerular permeability to albumin in recurrent focal segmental glomerulosclerosis. *N Eng J Med. 334*, 878-883 (1996).

[99] Srivastava T, Garola RE, Kestila M, Garola RE, Kestila M, Tryggvason K, Ruotsalainen V, Sharma M, Savin VJ, Jalanko H, Warady BA. Recurrence of proteinuria following renal transplantation in congenital nephrotic syndrome of the Finnish type. *Pediatr Nephrol. 21,* 711-718 (2006).

[100] Zenker M, Aigner T, Wendler O, Tralau, Muntefering H, Fenski R, Pitz S, Schumacher V, Royer-Pokora B, Wuhl E, Cochat P, Bouvier R, Kraus C, Mark K, Madlon H, Dotsch J, Rascher W, Maruniak-Chudek, Lennert T, Neumann LM, Reis A. Human Laminin beta 2 deficieny causes congenital nephrosis with mesengial sclerosis and distinct eye abnormalities. *Hum Mol Genet. 13*, 2625-2632 (2004).

[101] Shih NY, Li J, karpitskii V, Nguyen A, Dustin ML, kanagawa O, Miner JH, Shaw AS. Congenital nephrotic syndrome in mice lacking CD associated protein. *Science. 286,* 312-315 (1999).

[102] Dreyer SD, Zhou G, Baldini A, Winterpacht A, Zabel B, Cole W, Johnson RL, Lee B. Mutations in LMX1B cause abnormal skeletal patterning and renal dysplasia in nail patella syndrome. *Nat Genet. 19,* 47-50 (1998).

[103] Heeringa SF, Chernin G, Chaki M, Zhou W, Sloan AJ, Ji Z, Xie LX, Salviati L, Hurd TW, Vega-Warner V, Killen PD, Raphael Y, Ashraf S, Ovunc B, Schoeb DS, McLaughlin HM, Airik R, Vlangos CN, Gbadegesin R, Hinkes B, Saisawat P, Trevisson E, Doimo M, Casarin A, Pertegato V, Giorgi G, Prokisch H, Rötig A, Nürnberg G, Becker C, Wang S, Ozaltin F, Topaloglu R, Bakkaloglu A, Bakkaloglu SA, Müller D, Beissert A, Mir S, Berdeli A, Varpizen S, Zenker M, Matejas V, Santos-Ocaña C, Navas P, Kusakabe T, Kispert A, Akman S, Soliman NA, Krick S, Mundel P, Reiser J, Nürnberg P, Clarke CF, Wiggins RC, Faul C, Hildebrandt F. COQ6 mutations in human patients produce nephrotic syndrome with sensorineural deafness. *J Clin Invest. 121,* 2013-2014 (2011).

In: Handbook of Genitourinary Medicine: New Research   ISBN: 978-1-62618-226-4
Editor: Rashmi R. Singh   © 2013 Nova Science Publishers, Inc.

Chapter IX

Epigenetic Modifications in Urooncology

Muzeyyen Izmirli[1], Davut Alptekin[2] and Ulkan Kilic[1]
[1]Bezmialem Vakif University, Medical School,
Department of Medical Biology, Istanbul, Turkey
[2]Cukurova University, Medical School,
Department of Medical Biology,
Adana, Turkey

Abstract

Epigenetics including small, noncoding RNAs, DNA modifications and histone modifications is heritable changes in gene expression. It refers to functional modifications of the genome, but does not involve any changes in the nucleotide sequence. Cancer is the uncontrolled growth of abnormal cells in the body.

Both genetic and epigenetic alterations play a key role in cancer development. Epigenetic modifications influence gene silencing, which is important virtually for all steps in carcinogenesis including cancer initiation, progression, invasion and metastatis. Epigenetic modifications as molecular markers are being extensively explored for cancer risk evaluation, early detection, prognosis stratification, and treatment response prediction in urooncology, including prostate, bladder, renal, ovarian and endometrial cancers.

Due to epigenetic alterations are pharmacologically reversible, which makes them an attractive target in cancer therapeutics. For cancer screening and detection, tumor methylation biomarkers are useable at predicting prognosis via the assessment of markers in body fluids such as ascites, serum or plasma.

In this chapter, we discuss the main epigenetic changes related to carcinogenesis and urogenital cancer biomarkers.

Introduction

The most common feature of epigenetic mechanisms is that they are heritable between mother and daughter cells and also between generations [1]. The main interest of epigenetic is how cells and organisms with identical DNA have such phenotypic differences. Alterations in environmental factors (i.e. geographical differences such as altitude, flora, and weather conditions) and dietary compounds can shuffle the level of epigenetic organizing, and therefore epigenetic mechanisms are able to affect the risk of the diseases [2]. Thus, individual differences in the relationship between disease, healing and progress of disease are of subject of the epigenetic [1].

The key point of epigenetics is the fact that epigenetic factors do not affect the original sequence of DNA. Epigenetic factors mentioned above affect silencing of the genes and virtually all cancer pathways including different stages such as initiation, progression, invasion and metastasis. Epigenetic mechanisms involved in DNA modification, histone modifications and small, noncoding RNAs. DNA methylation which suppresses the gene expression is one of the well known. The second epigenetic mechanism, histone modifications, affects chromatin remodeling and subsequently causes active or repressed transcription factors of genes. The other mechanism which is small noncoding RNA [small interfering RNA (siRNA), microRNA (miRNA)] can induce the methylation of the promoter, therefore silencing the gene [3].

Cancer is a disease characterized by unregulated cell growing. Cell cleavage in an unregulated manner ultimately results in abnormal proliferation, differentiation and cell death. Moreover, these cells are transported throughout the body via lymphatic system or bloodstream. Urogenital system cancer comprises endometrial, ovarian, prostate, kidney and bladder, cancers etc. Urogenital cancers involve in a multi-step process that accumulates alterations, genetic or epigenetic [4].

Epigenetic modifications promise novel biomarkers for early cancer detection, prediction, prognosis, and response to treatment. Furthermore, reversal of epigenetic changes represents a potential target of novel therapeutic strategies and medication design. There has been an explosion of data and studies published in the last decade regarding the epigenetic mechanisms and their involvement in the development of phenotypes and diseases [5].

The current section aims to provide an introduction to the field of epigenetics, with examples of the most interesting studies related to this topic. In this chapter, some of the main epigenetic changes and related biomarkers that have been associated with urogenital cancer are summarized.

Epigenetics

In 1942, the conception of epigenetics was put forward by Conrad Hal Waddington, focused on the embryology field, using studies in *Drosophila melanogaster* [6]. Epigenetics is characterized as heritable changes in gene expression that are not due to modification in the sequence of DNA [7]. The important epigenetic modifications include the mechanisms that control the DNA sequence directly or indirectly. As mentioned above, the key point of epigenetic is the fact that epigenetic factors do not affect the original sequence of DNA which is reversible and heritable. Epigenetics also play a fundamental role in biological diversity such as phenotypic variation among genetically identical individuals [8], enabling cells to have distinct identities although containing the same genetic information. The most common phenomens that are classified as epigenetic changes are DNA modifications, histone modifications and small, noncoding RNAs [9].

Indirect Control of DNA

This is the first mechanism involving the posttranscriptional modifications. This epigenetic mechanism stops the function of mRNA and therefore inhibits protein synthesis using small and noncoding RNAs [4].

Noncoding RNAs

Indirect control mechanism of DNA sequence includes posttranscriptional modifications such as miRNAs, siRNA. The well known non-coding RNA is miRNA which has around 22 nucleotides that are coded by long non-coding RNA or introns of genes. miRNAs are transcribed in the nucleus and undergo several modifications prior to their maturation. miRNA and siRNA are both processed by the same machinery and use similar or identical protein complexes [10].

miRNA can inhibit translation of mRNA into protein by three ways. Firstly, if the miRNA is a direct sequence complement of the mRNA, the miRNA binds to the mRNA sequence, then the RNA interference (RNAi) pathway is triggered, and the target mRNA is degraded and finally the RNA-induced silencing complex (RISC complex) is activated. Secondly, if the miRNA is not suitable to match with the mRNA, the miRNA partially binds to the 3' untranslated region (UTR) of the mRNA and interferes the actions of target mRNA. Thirdly, miRNAs could regulate gene transcription by targeting promoter-associated ncRNAs [10-14].

Direct Control of DNA

This is the second mechanism that involves DNA (DNA methylation) and chromatin (histone acetylation, methylation, phosphorylation, s-nitrosylation, ubiquitination and sumoylation) modifications [4].

DNA Modifications

DNA modifications include covalent DNA modification, noncovalent DNA modification, and feed forward otoregulation by transcriptional factors. The best studied DNA modification is methylation of DNA that includes X chromosome inactivation, genome imprinting, and silencing of transposons and other parasitic elements [15].

DNA methylation (covalent DNA modification), an enzymatic reaction that occurs after DNA replication, is a type of covalent chemical modification in which binding of a methyl group at the carbon 5 position of the cytosine ring in CpG dinucleotides exists [16]. DNA methyltransferases (DNMTs) transfer methyl groups from S-adenosylmethionine to C the CpG nucleotide.

There are four types of DNA methyltransferases (DNMTs), including DNMT1, DNMT3A, DNMT3B, and DNMT3L. DNMTs control the degree of methylation of the genome; for instance DNMT1 is responsible for the phase maintenance of methylation. During S phase of DNA replication, DNMT1 is required for organizing the activity level of DNMTs. DNMT1 contains functional regions which are N-terminal and C-terminal ends. N-terminal region includes a cysteine-rich HRX-like region and a repetitious lysine-glycine part. The functional regions of DNMTs are required for DNMTs interaction with proliferating cell nuclear antigen, which is adjacent to the nuclear localization signal. C-terminal region is an active site which is called 'red box' [17]. DNMT3A and DNMT3B play a role in de novo methylation for creating the methylation pattern necessary during embryonic development. These two members of the DNMT family are highly expressed in embryonic stem cells and down-regulated in differentiated cells [18].

Although the DNMT3L does not have enzymatic activity, it regulates the activity of the other methyltransferases [19].

There are two recommended mechanisms for methylation to inhibit gene expression. In direct inhibition; the methylated chromosome holds back transcription by blocking the approach of the transcriptases. The second method is indirect inhibition; in which two types of protein, methylation-binding proteins (MBDs) and histone deacetylase (HDAC) are amended to the chromosome [20]. MBDs are present in transcription co-repressor complexes, described as MeCP2, MBD1 and MBD2. These are nonhomologous that can interact with other gene repressing mechanisms involving other members of the epigenetic machinery such as HDAC and histone methyltransferases (HMT).

As a consequence, chromatin reconfiguration and gene silencing exist [21]. MBD1 is able to bind unmethylated DNA via its third C-C zinc-finger motif. MBD2 has a characteristic stretch of glycine and arginine residues in the MBD domain, which when these are mutated, prevent the binding of MBD to methylated CpGs in mammals [5]. Unmethylated CpG islands generate a chromatin structure during optimal gene expression.

A special protein, CXXC finger protein 1 (CFP1), related with unmethylated CpG islands is associated with HMT that creates domains rich in the histone methylation [22].

DNA methylation level is not stable for different types of tissues. The alterations in the level of DNA methylation for a special type of any tissue are called 'abnormal levels of methylation'. The abnormal DNA methylation levels are hypermethylation and hypomethylation. Moreover, the level of methylation changes during the growth of human beings and the development of diseases.

Normally, about 50% of the CpG islands, which customarily are located in the promoter region of housekeeping genes, are unmethylated and thus are active. When those CpGs become methylated, the corresponding gene is silenced. On the other hand, CPGs that are located elsewhere in genes do not influence transcription when they are methylated [23-25].

Hypermethylation of CpG islands in the promoter region of a gene can result in transcriptional silencing of the gene, and finally loss of protein expression. Therefore, hypermethylation of tumor suppressor genes causes gene-silencing [26]. DNA methylation changes the biophysical properties of DNA. These changes can positively or negatively impresses the connective abilities of DNA and certain proteins.

For instance, if RNA poylmerase I is unable to bind to DNA correctly, then the process of transcribing DNA into RNA is altered. Many factors such as X-ray irradiation, temperature, smoking, folic acid deficiency affect the methylation level [27-28]. Hypermethylation of genes involved in the cell cycle, DNA repair, angiogenesis, apoptosis, and cell-cell interaction are involved in carcinogenesis.

In fact, during normal conditions, DNA hypermethylation occurs as a normal physiologic process. For instance the hypermethylation and thus inactivation of the second X chromosome result in the formation of the Barr body in females [10].

Chromatin Modifications

These modifications include both covalent and noncovalent modifications. Chromatin modifications in addition to the alterations in methylation levels result in silencing of the genes. Covalent chromatin modifications include histone acetylation, methylation, phosphorylation, s-nitrosylation, ubiquitination and sumoylation. Noncovalent chromatin modifications consist of histone exchange, histone heredity, fixing of the chromatin, chromatin interacting with noncoding RNA, and some other agents such as viruses, different proteins and long distance chromosome fields [3].

DNA packaged together with proteins including histones is called as chromatin. Histones comprise a globular C-terminal domain and N-terminal tail [29]. As N-terminal region of histones is changed, chromatin modifications occur as posttranslational modifications. Deacetylated histones contribute to a strict configuration of the DNA packaging. When an acetyl group is added on the N-terminal tail of the histones, DNA becomes less rigid due to negatively charged histones [30]. Histon modifications correspondingly affect chromatin conformation, gene transcription, DNA repair, DNA replication, and cell cycle checkpoints [31].

Histone is ticked via acetylated histone H3, and especially di or trimethylated histone H3 lysine 4 (H3K4me2, H3K4me3). For histone H3, methylation has been observed at multiple lysine sites, including H3K4, K9, K27, K36, and K79, and the addition of up to three methyl groups at each lysine produces a total of four methylation states: unmethylated, monomethylated, dimethylated, or trimethylated. H3K4 trimethylation (H3K4me3) is strongly associated with transcriptional competence and activation, with the highest levels observed near transcriptional start sites (TSS) [19].

The best known histone modification is the acetylation of the lysine residue. Histone acetylation is associated with transcriptional activation whereas deacetylation is linked with transcriptional repression like the other histone modifications.

The end of the acetylation lysine residue is positively charged in the histone tail, reducing the tight of the bond between the histone tails and DNA. This process opens up the DNA/histone complex such that it is accessible to transcription factors [32]. The other histone modification, the methylation, can affect transcription [10]. Alterations in the abundance of "linker" histones have been associated with chromatin configuration [33]. As mentioned above, distinct modifications play positive or negative roles on histones [34].

Histone modifications are catalyzed by many enzymes such as HMTs, histone demethylases (HDMs) histone acetyltransferases (HATs), and HDACs. HMTs add methyl groups to lysine or arginine residues in histones, while HDMs get rid of the methyl groups. HATs add acetyl groups to the lysine residues of histones, whereas HDACs are responsible for the removal of these groups [35]. Any abnormality in the HATs and HDACs activity trigger carcinogenesis processes [36].

Nucleosome Positions in Chromatin Remodeling

Not only alterations in the location in nucleosome but also modifications in their chemical and compositional features play key roles at genome regulation. Misregulation of nucleosome positioning as a result of many external stimuli leads to developmental defects and cancer [37].

Nucleosomes are normally situated canonical positions around promoter regions and random positions in gene sites [38]. The 5′ and 3′ ends of the genes present nucleosome-free regions. The presence or absence of nucleosomes in such regulatory regions determines the possibility of gene activation [39-40].

The nucleosome remodeling and deacetylase (NuRD) complex affect aberrant repression of target genes. Moreover, the translocation premyelocytic leukemia-retinoic acid receptor a (PML-RARa) represses gene transcription through several distinct mechanisms, including histone deacetylation, DNA methylation, histone modification, chromatin compaction, and heterochromatinization [41].

Another protein complex in nucleosome positioning is the switch/sucrose non fermentable (SWI/SNF) complex. These proteins target promoter regions and play positive or negative role via three biochemical pathways including nucleosome remodeling, nucleosome sliding, and octamer transfer [42-45].

Loss of Imprinting

Imprinted genes consist of nearly 1% of autosomal genes, possesses mono allelic expression, that is, only one copy of genes derived from one of the parents is present. DNA methylation and histone acetylation determine the imprinted genes. Gene expression depends on exclusively one parent [46]. Loss of imprinting causes of bi-allelic expression of the gene, or both copies are not expressed for gene dosage [32]. Imprinted genes are associated with many developmental diseases including Angelman syndrome, Prader-Willi syndrome, and Beckwith-Wiedemann syndrome. Additionally, this modification is related with bipolar disorder, autism, schizophrenia, and Tourette's syndrome in some cases [46].

Cancer

Cancer is a complex disease including multi step process that accumulates alterations. In cancer, cells divide and grow uncontrollably and invade nearby parts of the body. Genetic or epigenetic alteration play key role for cancer development [47]. Moreover, cancer connected with genetic and epigenetic modifications can be influenced by environmental and dietary factors. Especially, nicotine, radiation, lack of physical activity, obesity, environmental compounds and inorganic contaminants can change the epigenome, and can cause of the development of abnormalities [48-49].

Epigenetic aberrations are well established in the development and progression of cancer and their gradual accumulation is associated with advancing disease stage and grade [50].

DNA Methylation and Cancer

Since 1983, researchers have focused on methylation. As explained before, the appropriate DNA methylation within CpG dinucleotide islands plays a significant role in the regulation of gene. Aberrant methylation affects some mechanisms including tumor cell specific promoters, cell cycle, apoptosis, DNA repair mechanisms following the aberrances of differentiation and adhesion of cells [17].

The most studied epigenetic modification is DNA methylation in cancer. There are two methylation processes, are global DNA hypomethylation and promoter DNA hypermethylation, are observed in cancer cells.

Hypermethylation of the promoter region of tumor suppressor genes is associated with transcriptional silencing [51]. DNA hypomethylation is described in several tumor types such as prostate cancer, head-neck cancer [52-54]. Aberrant DNA methylation is widely accepted as a common mechanism used by tumor cells to silence tumor suppressor genes [50]. Lots of data has been published in different tumor types. For example; cell cycle (p14 and p16), signal transduction (Ras association domain family member 1; RASSF1A), DNA repair (O6-methylguanine-DNA methyltransferase; MGMT, mut L homolog 1; hMLH1), trombospondin 1 (TSP-1), and insulin like growth factor 2 (IGF2) [19, 57]. Tumor suppressor gene is high in normal 1 (HIN-1), H-cadherin (CDH13), recombinant interleukin (RIL), RASSF1A, and retinoic acid receptor 2 (RARβ2) were frequently methylated in both primary and metastatic tissues [58].

Dysfunction of DNA repairs genes, such as hMLH1 (DNA mismatch repair protein) and MGMT associated with a microsatellite instability phenotype and can be an early event in the development of cancer [59-60]. Reduced cell cycle control can be involved with silencing of the cyclin dependent kinase inhibitor 2A (CDKN2A) gene and E-cadherin 1 (CDH1) gene is changed in cell migration and invasion [61].

The silenced promoter DNA hypermethylation of noncoding transcription yields associate with miRNAs. Overexpression of DNMTs has been linked to loss of miRNA expression in cancer [50].

Histon Modifications and Cancer

Histone modifications may underlie aberrant gene silencing in cancer. Kouzarides and colleagues have identified there are various types of histone tail modifications, such as acetylation, methylation, phosphorylation, ubiquitination. These modifications have ability to enhance or block transcription factor binding. Whereupon, transcriptionally active euchromatin and inactive heterochromatin are exist [69].

The differentiation of HDACs enzyme system has been described in cancer development, and the level of HDAC expression can be change in cancer stage [70-72]. The HAT expression level has also been correlated with cancer [73]. Moreover, HDACs and DNMTs can be managed by miRNA; the all epigenetic system acts in conjunction to induce the chromatin conformation [19]. Chromatin modifying complexes, DNA methylation, and Polycomb (PcG) complexes and their contents are actively being pursued for their link to abnormal gene silencing in cancer. Moreover, SWI/SNF complexes, which mediates ATP-dependent chromatin remodeling processes, is chromatin modifying complexes and alters the position of nucleosomes along DNA [74-75].

Small Noncoding RNA and Cancer

Small none coding, single stranded RNAs called microRNAs (miRNAs), epigenetic phenomenon is posttranscriptional gene down regulation [77-78]. Although miRNAs are vital on normal cell physiology, their misexpression has been linked to cancer development, and miRNA profiles have been used to classify human cancers [79].

Individual miRNA can regulate about 200 targets, and one miRNA can control numerous biological or pathological signaling pathways by affecting the expressions and functions of their targets [80-82]. They target at the binding sites located mostly in the 30 untranslated regions (UTR) of mRNAs, and cause of mRNA degradation or translational repression [83].

miRNAs can also play important roles in carcinogenesis including angiogenesis, apoptosis, metastasis. The miRNA-17-92 was the first oncogenic miRNAs, is called oncomir [84]. Oncogenic miRNAs includes a number of members, such as miRNA-17, miRNA-18, miRNA-19a, miRNA-19b-1, miRNA-20a, miRNA-21, and miRNA-92-1 [85]. miRNA-221, miRNA -222, miRNA-223, p27 (Kip1), are associated with various cancerous conditions [86-87]. The well studied miRNAs is also let-7 family has been shown to be regulated by DNA promoter methylation [88-92]. MiRNA-15a and miRNA-16-1 are tumor suppressor miRNAs. They target the expression of the anti-apoptotic protein Bcl-2, thereby promoting apoptosis [93]. Another tumor suppressor miRNA-122 targets disintegrin and metalloprotease which are known promoter of metastasis. miRNA-122 effects tumor angiogenesis and cancer cell invasion which are inhibited [94]. miRNA-126 also appears to inhibit cancer cell growth, proliferation, adhesion, and invasion, and is down-regulated in cancers [95]. Examples of some other oncogenic miRNAs include miRNA-10b, miRNA-372, miRNA-373, and examples of some other tumor suppressor miRNAs, include miRNA-34, miRNA-335, miRNA-143, miRNA-145, and miRNA-181a/b/c [96-98].

It is shown that miRNA profiles in cancer downregulation of tumor suppressor miRNAs (miRNA-206, miRNA-17-5p, miRNA-125a, miRNA-125b, miRNA-200, miRNA-34, and miRNA-31) and the overexpression of certain oncogenic miRNAs (miRNA-155, miRNA-10b, miRNA-373, and miRNA-520c), along with their correlation in cancer pathways and metastasis [99]. On the other hand, polymorphisms in miRNAs and their target sequences have been linked to variations in drug activation and metabolism, revealing the potential use of miRNA in pharmacogenomics [100].

Urogenital Cancers and Epigenetic Mechanisms

Urogenital cancers include prostate, bladder, ovarian, endometrial, kidney and testis cancers. In this section, prostate, bladder, ovarian, endometrial, kidney cancers are assessed for epigenetic mechanisms.

Prostate Cancer

Human prostate cancer is one of the most common cancer types and the second significant cancer killer of men in America. Epigenetic mechanisms affect the progression of prostate cancer [101].

Aberrant genomic distribution and level of histone modifications, nucleosome remodeling at the promoter-enhancer regions of the gene and androgen receptor (AR) mediated chromosomal looping may lead to the silencing of tumor suppressor genes and the activation of proto-oncogenes [102]. The acetylation of histone H3 (H3Ac) affects CRE-binding protein (CBP) and p300 which is AR coactivators, is increased in the prostate cancer cell line [103]. The methylation of histone H3K9 mono, di and tri methylation (H3K9me1, H3K9me2 and H3K9me3) has been connected with repression of AR target genes in prostate cancer cell lines.

In this mechanism, silencing of H3K9me1, H3K9me2 and H3K9me3 demethylases attracts the Lysine Specific Demethylase (LSD1), jmjc Domain Containing Histone Demethylase 2A and 2C (JHDM2A and JMJD2C, respectively) [102]. In prostate cancer, H3K4 methylations facilitate activation of proto-oncogene and increased repressive histone marks and lead to tumor suppressor gene silencing.

Furthermore, H3K27me3 genomic distribution change during prostate cancer progression and affects some tumor suppressor genes (growth arrest specific; GAS2, phosphatidylinositol 4,5 bisphosphate 3 kinase catalytic subunit gamma; PIK3CG and β-2 adrenergic receptor; ADRB2) for cancer development, cell growth, survival and invasion [104]. The increased level of the H3K27me3 brings about overexpression of enhancer of zeste 2 (EZH2) in prostate cancer [105-106]. Downregulation of EZH2 reactivates expression of some H3K27me3 target genes, resulting in prostate cancer cell cycle block and apoptosis [107]. It is shown that the levels of H3 lysine 18acetylation (H3K18Ac), H3K4me2 and H3K4me3 are independent predictors of prostate carcinoma recurrence in patients with low-grade tumors [108].

Hypermethylation is also responsible for the inactivation of some genes such as adenomatous polyposis coli (APC), CDH1, multi drug resistance 1 (MDR1) and RASSF1A in prostate cancer [109-111].

Moreover, hypermethylation correlated with tazarotene induced gene 1 (TIG1) and glutathione S-transferase M1 (GSTP1) genes are relationship between the pathologic stage and Gleason score and prostate cancer [102].

miRNAs may function as oncogenes or tumor suppressors [112]. Overexpression of the oncomers epigenetically silences the apoptosis related genes and induces tumor growth, invasion and metastasis. The altered expressions of some selected miRNAs are useful as biomarkers for diagnosis, prognosis, and classification of prostate cancer [113-114]. miRNA-200 family includes two groups which are situated on chromosome 1 and 12. The first group encodes miRNA-200b, miRNA-200a, and miRNA -429, and the second group encodes miRNA-200c and miRNA-141 [115]. It is found that there is relationship between miRNA -221, miRNA -222 and development, metastasis of prostate cancer [116].

Another potential oncomirs are miRNA-21 and miRNA-101, are overexpressed in solid tumors of prostate cancer [117]. miRNA-125b and miRNA-126 are important for cell proliferation and are found to be overexpressed in prostate cancer.

On the other hand, loss of tumor suppressor miRNAs is another mechanism related to the progression of prostate cancer [118-119]. In PC3 cells, expression of miRNA -146a resulted in remarkably reduced cell migration, invasion, proliferation, antiapoptosis and metastasis via silencing rho-associated coiled coil containing protein kinas 1(ROCK1) and then inhibiting the ROCK1 pathway [120].

In addition, miRNA-330 negatively correlates with the level of transcription factor E2F1 leading to the activation of apoptosis through suppression of Akt signaling pathway in prostate cancer [121]. Involvement of p53 in miRNA-34a/, miRNA-34c-mediated apoptosis influence AR in prostate cancer cells [122].

Renal Cancer

In 2012, renal cancer is approximately 3 percent in America [101]. It is cited after mentioned that about epigenetic mechanisms associated with renal carcinoma. This type of the cancer also needs early detection using genetic and epigenetic biomarkers. Many epigenetic states are closely relationship between renal cancers.

Silencing due to DNA methylation of a number of genes may play a role in renal carcinogenesis. These are the p53-inducible gene 14-3-3 sigma, drug resistance gene (ABCG2), a gap junction molecule connexin 32, actin-binding protein DAL-1/4.1B, tissue inhibitor metalloproteinase 3 (TIMP3), the fragile histidine triad (FHIT) gene, cell adhesion molecule junction plakoglobin (JUP), HGF activator inhibitor HAI-2, a member of the homeobox gene family (HOXB13), tissue-specific proapoptotic BH3- only protein BCL2-interacting killer (BIK), TU3A (tumor suppressor gene) and XAF1 which antagonizes the anticaspase activity of X-linked inhibitor of apoptosis (XIAP) [123-135].

Moreover, RASSF1, twist homolog 1 (TWIST1), paired-like homeodomain 2 (PITX2), CDH13, heparan sulfate 3-O -sulfotransferase 2 (HS3ST2), T-cell acute lymphocytic leukemia 1 (TAL1), Wilms' tumor 1 (WT1), matrix metallopeptidase 2 (MMP2), islet cell autoantigen 1 (ICA1) and tumor suppressor candidate 3 (TUSC3), the gamma-aminobutyric acid A receptor beta 3 (GABRB3) genes are more frequently methylated in sporadic renal cancers [136].

DNA hypermethylation and repressive histone modification have been observed in the secreted frizzled-related protein 1 (SFRP1), SFRP2, SFRP5, WNT inhibitory factor 1 (WIF1) and dickkopf homolog 3 (DKK3) genes [137]. Hypermethylation of the ubiquitin carboxyl-terminal esterase L1 (UCHL1) gene, involving in the regulation of cellular ubiquitin levels plays important roles in different cellular process, and transforming growth factor beta receptor III (TGFBR3) cause gene silencing and this process correlated with poor outcome in renal cancer [138]. Additionally, promoter hypermethylation of CDKN2A, HOXB13 and CDH13 are present in renal cancer.

Additionally, the methylated identified genes are SFRP1, RASSF1A, keratin 19 (KRT19), chemokine ligand 16 (CXCL16), basonuclin1 (BNC1), PDZ and LIM domain 4 (PDLIM4), reprimo (RPRM), cystatin 6 (CST6), insulin like growth factor binding protein 3 (IGFBP3), gremlin 1 (GREM1), sodium channel voltage gated type Beta I (SCNN1B), synaptotagmin-6 (SYT6), dachshund homolog 1 (DACH1), transcription factor AP-2 alpha (TFAP2A), collagen type XIV alpha 1 (COL14A1) and COL15A1 in renal cancer [123, 138].

On the other hand, hypomethylated a number of genes affect renal carcinogenesis. These are Carbonic Anhydrase IX (CA9) gene (transmembrane glycoprotein), SET domain containing 2 (SETD2) gene and the LSD-5C gene [123, 139]. Lower levels of H3K4me2, H3K9me2 and H3K18 acetylation are reported to predict poorer prognosis in renal cancer [134].

There are a lot of studies about another epigenetic mechanism miRNA. Downregulation of miRNA-141 and miRNA-200c and upregulation of miRNA-210 in renal cancer compared to normal renal parenchymal tissue. miRNA-141 and miRNA-200c can inhibit epithelial mesenchymal transition (EMT) protein which represses E-cadherin by indirectly and effects the development of renal cancer [140-141].

Bladder Cancer

In America, bladder cancer is the frequencies of the 3 percent in all cancer types in 2012 [101]. Different epigenetic mechanism including DNA modification, histone modification and non coding RNA, has been reported in bladder cancer [19]. However, there is limited data on epigenetic modifications in bladder cancer.

Silencing due to DNA hypermethylation of a number of genes may play a role in bladder carcinogenesis. These are lysyl oxidase like 1-4 (LOXL1 and LOXL4), COL1A2 which affect E-cadherin expression, COL1A, GSTP1, IGFBP, CDKN2A, TWIST1, RARβ2, MMP11, fibroblast growth factor 18 (FGF18), retinoblastoma (Rb), Methylguanine-DNA Methyltransferase (MGMT), Laminin-5 (LN5), nidogen 2 (NID2) and runt related transcription factor 3 (RUNX3) genes [142-147].

For the histone modification, histone H3lysine9 methylation has been associated with aberrant gene silencing in the T24 bladder tumor cell line [148].

Endometrial Cancer

Endometrial cancer (EC) is the most common gynaecological malignancy affecting women in the western world. EC is affected many gene which is silenced different epigenetic mechanisms [149]. The frequency of the EC is 3 percent in America in 2012 [101].

DNA methylation affects genes encoding tumor suppressors, apoptosis inhibitors, cell cycle regulators, steroid receptors, transcription factors, angiogenesis modulators and oncoproteins in ECs. Specifically, a high frequency of methylation in tumors and cell lines has been reported for APC, caspase 8 (CASP8), CDH1, ERa-promoter-C, hMLH1, PR-promoter-B, RASSF1A, thrombospondin 2 (THBS2), CDKN2A, p73 and phosphatase and tensin homolog (PTEN). Promoter hypermethylation of the period-1 gene (PER1) have been found in EC, recommending a role for circadian rhythms in EC development [150-153]. In addition, epigenetics affects the steroid receptor cascades in EC. Silencing of estrogen receptor (ER), transcription factor-encoding PAX2, homeoboxA1 (HOXA10) and HOXA11 by aberrant DNA methylation occurs in EC [149]. DNA methylation associates with microsatellite instability (MSI) in ECs. DNA mutations in MSI-related mismatch repair genes, are hMLH1, MGMT, Werner syndrome (WRN) and breast cancer 1 (BRCA1) genes, cause transcriptional silencing. Methylation of the sestrin 3 (SESN3), thyroid transcription factor 1 (TITF1), SFRP1 and SFRP4 genes cause MSI, and associate with EC [154].

Mutated miRNAs are common in EC. EC upregulated miRNAs typically include proapoptotic gene products (miRNA-96, -150, -185, -186 and -513a-5p). Downregulated miRNAs consist of targeting metastasis promoters (miRNA-1, -193, -455-5p and -765) and antiapoptotic transcripts (miRNA-26, -133, -196, -377 and -542-3p/5p). The tumor suppressor forkheadbox O1 (FOXO1) is cooperatively downregulated by miRNA-9, -27, -96, -153, -182, -183 and -186 in EC cells.

Furthermore, the overexpressed miRNA-186 and -150 affect some protein, which are the proapoptotic, ATP binding receptor P2X7 in EC tumors. miRNA-129-2 is silenced by histone deacetylation, this situation causes of upregulation of the oncogenic transcription factor SRY box containing gene 4 (SOX4), is miRNA-129-2's target [155-156]. For EC drug resistance and possible cancer stemness, some data are shown that there are many miRNAs including the upregulated miRNA-155, -182, -185 and the downregulated miRNA-30c, -101, -455-5p and -518c. Another well known tumor suppressive miRNA-200c, mediates chemosensitivity of aggressive EC cell lines [155].

Ovarian Cancer

Ovarian carcinoma is the most lethal gynecological cancer in 2012. In America, ovarian cancer is the frequencies of the 6 percent in all cancer types [101]. Just as in the case of all cancer types, for ovarian cancer, there is also a need for early detection biomarkers. For this purpose, some studies shown that altered epigenetic states are closely relationship between ovarian tumorigenesis.

Ovarian cancer tumor progression is well characterized by a number of combinatorial epigenetic modifications. Methylated RASSF1A, H-Sulf-1, BRCA1, APC, DAPK, CDKN2A and HOXA10 genes are exist. A number of genes, including the classical tumor suppressors (BRCA1, p16, RASSF1A and MLH1), imprinted genes [adrenodoxin reductase homolog (ARH1)], proapoptotic genes [pleimorphic adenoma gene like 1 (LOT1), death associated protein kinase 1 (DAPK), target of methylation induced silencing (TMS1/ASC), and prader willi region 4 (PAR-4)] and cell adhesion genes (ICAM-1 and CDH1), are hypermethylated and down-regulated in ovarian cancer [157-162].

In addition, the HSulf-1 gene acts on cell surface heparin sulfate proteoglycans and inhibit growth factor signaling and angiogenesis. Methylated HSulf-1 gene is found in over 50% of ovarian tumors and cell lines [163-164]. Moreover, the partner and localizer of BRCA2 (PALB2) and class III tubulin (TUBB3) genes have been reported to be hypermethylated in ovarian cancer [156, 165].

Recently, hypermethylated candidate tumor suppressor genes have been discovered in ovarian cancer. These are secreted protein acidic and rich in cysteine (SPARC), angiopoietin-like protein 2 (ANGPTL2), collagen and calcium binding EGF domains 1 (CCBE1), hypermethylated in cancer 1 (HIC1), CDH13, connective tissue growth factor (CTGF) and APC genes [19]. The indicators, such as HE4 and CA-125, remain highly informative, epigenetic markers could supplement these approaches, possibly increasing sensitivity and specificity sufficiently for early detection [123].

In ovarian cancer, there are hypomethylated IGF2, an imprinted gene implicated and claudin-4, whose overexpression leads to disrupted tight junctions between epithelial ovarian cells [166-167]. In addition to decreased methylation of LINE-1 elements has been correlated with ovarian cancer [168]. Hypomethylation and upregulation of the multi drug transporter (ABCG2) gene are also shown to occur during drug-acquired chemoresistance in ovarian carcinoma cell lines. Decreased methylation of the metastasis promoters including TUBB3, breast cancer specific protein 1 (SNCG), mammary serine protease inhibitor (MASPIN) and claudin 4 (CLDN4) occurs in late-stage ovarian cancers [160, 169-171].

Histone modifications regulate normal ovarian functions which are estrogen synthesis, folliculogenesis, and luteal phase activity [172]. For example, HDAC enzymes influence downregulate disintegrin and metalloprotease domain 19 (ADAM19) [173]. Loss of H3K27 trimethylation has also been associated with poor prognosis in ovarian cancer [174]. The overexpression of HDACs correlates with high-grade tumors and poor prognosis in ovarian cancer [175].

miRNAs including miRNA-199a, miRNA-200a, miRNA-214, miRNA-100, miRNA-214 and let-7i have been demonstrated to target the tumor suppressor and associate with regulation in ovarian cancer [80]. Moreover, miRNA-429, miRNA-200a, and miRNA-200b are found to be associated with ovarian malignancies [176]. Some miRNAs upregulate proapoptotic pathway and downregulate suppress of the metastasis in ovarian cancer. Upregulated miRNAs are miRNA-10a/b, -21, -130a, -221, -222 and -223, whereas down regulated miRNAs are tumor suppressors such as miRNA-9, -15a, -16, -34, -125, -155 and the let-7 family [177]. Additionally, methylation biomarkers can augment the CA-125 in ovarian cancer [176].

Clinical Application

Cancer can be detected by a number ways, including the presence of certain signs and symptoms, screening tests or medical imaging. On the other hand, cancer is usually treated with chemotherapy, radiation therapy and surgery. Epigenetic and genetic biomarkers are important instruments for diagnosis, prognosis and therapy of cancer. Epigenetic modifications as molecular markers are being extensively explored for cancer risk evaluation, early detection, prognosis stratification, and treatment response prediction in urooncology [19]. Due to epigenetic changes, including DNA methylation and histone modifications, are pharmacologically reversible, which makes them an attractive target in cancer therapeutics. For disease screening and detection, tumor methylation biomarkers are useable at predicting prognosis via assessment of markers in body fluids such as ascites, serum or plasma [123]. Moreover, the potential role of DNA methylation markers possesses more important for individual therapy, in medical care [5].

Despite fact that epigenetic drugs are usable, epigenetic monotherapies are not effective on its own activity against solid tumors. However, the combination of DNA demehylating agents with HDAC inhibitors therapies provides potentially safer therapeutic options [178]. The combination of both agents has a strong synergistic effect on the reactivation of silenced genes and antiproliferative on cancer cells.

Moreover, nucleoside and nonnucleoside analogs can be used to demethylate the gene of interest [123]. The DNMT inhibitors are mainly cytosine analogs: 5-azacytidine, 5-aza-2'-deoxycytidine, 5,6-dihydro-5-azacytidine and zebularine. These analogs are incorporated into the DNA in the original cytosine positions during DNA replication [5]. Thus, target gene is demethylated and silenced.

HDAC inhibitors which regulate histone deacetylation act on genes and gene expression are silenced. These inhibitors are more sensitive tumor cells than normal cells. A variety of naturally occurring or synthetic HDAC inhibitors have been characterized for antitumor activities. The most widely used HDAC inhibitor is trichostatin A (TSA), but it limited use in the clinic due to its high toxicity. Suberoylannilide hydroxamic acid (SAHA), romidepsin (also known as depsipeptide or FK228) and polycomb group components are the HDAC inhibitor approved by US FDA. They inhibit histone H3K27 methylation, and induce selective apoptotic cell death in cancer. Polyamine analogs are also successful in inhibition of the gene in cancer. One natural HDAC, psammaplin A (PsA) inhibit HDAC and DNA methyletransferase activities [178].

Conclusion

This chapter have exemplified the assessing of epigenetic mechanism in urogenital carcinogenesis and largely described related with "epigenetic", "genitourinary cancer" research literature. Consequently, epigenetic modifications drive carcinogenesis. Well understanding of epigenetic molecular mechanisms will facilitate therapy of the genitourinary cancers. New technologies will represent sensitive and specific biomarker and epigenetic target therapy. In also individual therapy, the development of epigenetic biomarker and epigenetic therapeutic are expected to complement the genitourinary cancer therapy.

References

[1] Waterland, R. A., Michels, K. B. Epigenetic epidemiology of the developmental origins hypothesis. *Annu. Rev. Nutr.* 2007; 27:363-88.

[2] Hardy, T., Tollefsbol, T. O. Epigenetic diet: impact on the epigenome and cancer. *Epigenomics.* 2011; 3(4):503-518.

[3] Bond, D. M., Finnegan, E. J. Passing the message on: inheritance of epigenetic traits. *Trends Plant Sci.* 2007; 12(5):211-6.

[4] Holliday, R. Epigenetics: a historical overview. *Epigenetics.* 2006; 1(2): 76-80.

[5] Li, X. Q., Guo, Y. Y., De, W. DNA methylation and microRNAas in cancer. *World J. Gastroenterol.* 2012; 18(9):882-888.

[6] Waddington, C. H. The epigenotype. *Endeavour.* 1942; 1:18–20.

[7] Martin, C., Zhang, Y. Mechanisms of epigenetic inheritance. *Curr. Opin. Cell Biol.* 2007; 19(3):266-72.

[8] Morgan, H. D., Sutherland, H. G., Martin, D. I., Whitelaw, E. Epigenetic inheritance at the agouti locus in the mouse. *Nat. Genet.* 1999; 23:314–318.

[9] Riddihough, G., Zahn, L. M. Epigenetics. What is epigenetics? Introduction. *Science.* 2010; 330:611.

[10] Hamilton, J. P. Epigenetics: Principles and Practice. *Digestive Diseases.* 2011; 29:130-135.

[11] Omoto, S., Fujii, Y. R. Regulation of human immunodeficiency virus 1 transcription by nef microRNA. *J. Gen. Virol.* 2005; 86:751–755.

[12] Gonzalez, S., Pisano, D. G., Serrano, M. Mechanistic principles of chromatin remodeling guided by siRNAs and miRNAs. *Cell Cycle.* 2008; 7:2601–2608.

[13] Bartel, D. P. MicroRNAs: target recognition and regulatory functions. *Cell.* 2009; 136:215–233.

[14] Grimson, A., Farh, K. K., Johnston, W. K., Garrett-Engele, P., Lim, L. P., Bartel, D. P. MicroRNA targeting specificity in mammals: determinants beyond seed pairing. *Mol. Cell.* 2007; 27:91–105.

[15] Mohn, F., Schubeler, D. Genetics and epigenetics: stability and plasticity during cellular differentiation. *Trends Genet.* 2009; 25:129-136.

[16] Zuo, T., Tycko, B., Liu, T. M., Lin, J. J., Huang, T. H. Methods in DNA methylation profiling. *Epigenomics.* 2009; 1:331-345.

[17] Esteller, M. Epigenetics in cancer. *N Engl. J. Med.* 2008; 358:1148-1159.

[18] Bird, A. P. CpG-rich islands and the function of DNA methylation. *Nature.* 1986; 321: 209-213.

[19] Brait, M., Sidransky, D. Cancer epigenetics: above and beyond. *ToxicolMech. Methods.* 2011; 21(4):275-288.

[20] Klose, R. J., Bird, A. P. Genomic DNA methylation: the mark and its mediators. *Trends Biochem. Sci.* 2006; 31:89–97.

[21] Nan, X., Ng, H. H., Johnson, C. A., Laherty, C. D., Turner, B. M., Eisenman, R. N., Bird, A. Transcriptional repression by the methyl-CpG-binding protein MeCP2 involves a histone deacetylase complex. *Nature.* 1998; 393:386–389.

[22] Portela, A., Esteller, M. Epigenetic modifications and human disease. *Nat. Biotechnol.* 2010; 28:1057–1068.

[23] Cedar, H., Bergman, Y. Linking DNA methylation and histone modification: patterns and paradigms. *Nat. Rev. Genet.* 2009; 10:295-304.

[24] Chang, S. C., Tucker, T., Thorogood, N. P., Brown, C. J. Mechanisms of X-chromosome inactivation. *Front Biosci.* 2006; 11:852-866.

[25] Bird, A. P. DNA methylation and the frequency of CpG in animal DNA. *Nucleic Acids Res.* 1980; 8:1499-1504.

[26] Herman, J. G., Baylin, S. B. Gene silencing in cancer in association with promoter hypermethylation. *N Engl. J. Med.* 2003; 349(21):2042–54.

[27] Cadieux, B., Ching, T. T., VandenBerg, S. R., Costello, J. F. Genome-wide hypomethylation in human glioblastomas associated with specific copy number alteration, methylenetetrahydrofolate reductase allele status, and increased proliferation. *Cancer Res.* 2006; 66:8469-8476.

[28] Goelz, S. E., Vogelstein, B., Hamilton, S. R., Feinberg, A. P. Hypomethylation of DNA from benign and malignant human colon neoplasms. *Science.* 1985; 228:187-190.

[29] Luger, K., Mader, A. W., Richmond, R. K., Sargent, D. F., Richmond, T. J. Crystal structure of the nucleosome core particle at 2.8 A resolution. *Nature.* 1997; 389:251–260.

[30] Struhl, K. Histone acetylation and transcriptional regulatory mechanisms. *Genes Dev.* 1998; 12:599–606.

[31] Sawan, C., Vaissiere, T., Murr, R., Herceg, Z. Epigenetic drivers and genetic passengers on the road to cancer. *Mutat. Res.* 2008; 642:1–13.

[32] Feinberg, A. P. Epigenetics at the epicenter of modern medicine. *JAMA.* 2008; 299: 1345–1350.

[33] Clapier, C. R., Cairns, B. R. The biology of chromatin remodeling complexes. *Annu. Rev. Biochem.* 2009; 78:273–304.

[34] Sharma, S., Kelly, T. K., Jones, P. A. Epigenetics in cancer. *Carcinogenesis.* 2010; 31: 27–36.

[35] Choudhuri, S., Cui, Y., Klaassen, C. D. Molecular targets of epigenetic regulation and effectors of environmental influences. *Toxicol. Appl. Pharmacol.* 2010; 245(3):378–393.

[36] Mottet, D., Castronovo, V. Histone deacetylases: target enzymes for cancer therapy. *Clin. Exp. Metastasis.* 2008; 25(2):183–189.

[37] Jiang, C., Pugh, B. F. A compiled and systematic reference map of nucleosome positions across the Saccharomyces cerevisiae genome. *Genome Biol.* 2009; 10:R109.

[38] Mavrich, T. N., Ioshikhes, I. P., Venters, B. J., Jiang, C., Tomsho, L. P., Qi, J., Schuster, S. C., Albert, I., Pugh, B. F. A barrier nucleosome model for statistical positioning of nucleosomes throughout the yeast genome. *Genome Res.* 2008; 18:1073–1083.

[39] Yuan, G. C., Liu, Y. J., Dion, M. F., Slack, M. D., Wu, L. F., Altschuler, S. J., Rando, O. J. Genome-scale identification of nucleosome positions in S. cerevisiae. *Science.* 2005; 309:626–630.

[40] Schones, D. E., Cui, K., Cuddapah, S., Roh, T. Y., Barski, A., Wang, Z., Wei, G., Zhao, K. Dynamic regulation of nucleosome positioning in the human genome. *Cell.* 2008; 132:887–898.

[41] Di Croce, L., Raker, V. A., Corsaro, M., Fazi, F., Fanelli, M., Faretta, M., Fuks, F., Lo Coco, F., Kouzarides, T., Nervi, C., Minucci, S., Pelicci, P. G. Methyltransferase recruitment and DNA hypermethylation of target promoters by an oncogenic transcription factor. *Science.* 2002; 295:1079–1082.

[42] Langst, G., Becker, P. B. Nucleosome remodeling: one mechanism, many phenomena? *Biochim. Biophys. Acta.* 2004; 1677:58–63.

[43] Segal, E., Fondufe-Mittendorf, Y., Chen, L., Taström, A., Field, Y., Moore, I. K., Wang, J. P., Widom, J. A genomic code for nucleosome positioning. *Nature.* 2006; 442: 772–778.

[44] Weissman, B., Knudsen, K. E. Hijacking the chromatin remodeling machinery: impact of SWI/SNF perturbations in cancer. *Cancer Res.* 2009; 69:8223–8230.

[45] Taby, R., Issa, J. P. Cancer epigenetics. *CA Cancer J. Clin.* 2010; 60:376–392.

[46] Jirtle, R. L., Skinner, M. K. Environmental epigenomics and disease susceptibility. *Nat. Rev. Genet.* 2007; 8:253–262.

[47] Kinzler, K. W., Vogelstein, B. Lessons from hereditary colorectal cancer. *Cell.* 1996; 87:159–170.

[48] Skinner, M. K., Guerrero-Bosagna, C. Environmental signals and transgenerational epigenetics. *Epigenomics.* 2009; 1(1):111–117.

[49] Jaenisch, R., Bird, A. Epigenetic regulation of gene expression: how the genome integrates intrinsic and environmental signals. *Nat. Genet.* 2003; 33:245–254.

[50] Jones, P. A., Baylin, S. B. The epigenomics of cancer. *Cell.* 2007; 128:683–692.

[51] Ventura, A., Jacks, T. MicroRNAs and cancer: short RNAs go a long way. *Cell.* 2009; 136:586–591.

[52] Feinberg, A. P., Vogelstein, B. Hypomethylation of ras oncogenes in primary human cancers. *Biochem. Biophys. Res. Commun.* 1983; 111: 47-54.

[53] Bedford, M. T., van Helden, P. D. Hypomethylation of DNA in pathological conditions of the human prostate. *Cancer Res.*1987; 47: 5274-5276.

[54] Smith, I. M., Mydlarz, W. K., Mithani, S. K., Califano, J. A. DNA global hypomethylation in squamous cell head and neck cancer associated with smoking, alcohol consumption and stage. *Int. J. Cancer.* 2007; 121:1724–1728.

[55] Simpson, A. J., Caballero, O. L., Jungbluth, A., Chen, Y. T., Old, L. J. Cancer/testis antigens, gametogenesis and cancer. *Nat. Rev. Cancer.* 2005; 5:615–625.

[56] Glazer, C. A., Smith, I. M., Ochs, M. F., Begum, S., Westra, W., Chang, S. S., Sun, W., Bhan, S., Khan, Z., Ahrendt, S., Califano, J. A. Integrative discovery of epigenetically derepressed cancer testis antigens in NSCLC. *PLoS ONE.* 2009; 4:e8189.

[57] Ehrlich, M. DNA hypomethylation in cancer cells. *Epigenomics.* 2009; 1:239-259.

[58] Feng, W., Orlandi, R., Zhao, N., Carcangiu, M. L., Tagliabue, E., Xu, J., Bast, R. C., Yu, Y. Tumor suppressor genes are frequently methylated in lymph node metastases of breast cancers. *BMC Cancer.* 2010; 10:378.

[59] Nakagawa, H., Nuovo, G. J., Zervos, E. E., Martin, E. W., Salovaara, R., Aaltonen, L. A., de la Chapelle, A. Age-related hypermethylation of the 5′ region of MLH1 in normal colonic mucosa is associated with microsatellite-unstable colorectal cancer development. *Cancer Res.* 2001; 61(19):6991-6995.

[60] Herman, J. G., Umar, A., Polyak, K., Graff, J. R., Ahuja, N., Issa, J. P., Markowitz, S., Willson, J. K., Hamilton, S. R., Kinzler, K. W., Kane, M. F., Kolodner, R. D., Vogelstein, B., Kunkel, T. A., Baylin, S. B. Incidence and functional consequences of hMLH1 promoter hypermethylation in colorectal carcinoma. *Proc. Natl. Acad. Sci. US.* 1998; 95:6870-6875.

[61] Graff, J. R., Gabrielson, E., Fujii, H., Baylin, S. B., Herman, J. G. Methylation patterns of the E-cadherin 5′ CpG island are unstable and reflect the dynamic, heterogeneous loss of Ecadherin expression during metastatic progression. *J. Biol. Chem.* 2000; 275:2727-2732.

[62] Bachman, K. E., Herman, J. G., Corn, P. G., Merlo, A., Costello, J. F., Cavanee, W. K., Baylin, S. B., Graff, J. R. Methylation-associated silencing of the tissue inhibitor of metalloproteinase-3 gene suggest a suppressor role in kidney, brain, and other human cancers. *Cancer Res.* 1999; 59:798-802.

[63] Suzuki, H., Watkins, D. N., Jair, K. W., Schuebel, K. E., Markowitz, S. D., Chen, W. D., Pretlow, T. P., Yang, B., Akiyama, Y., Van Engeland, M., Toyota, M., Tokino, T., Hinoda, Y., Imai, K., Herman, J. G., Baylin, S. B. Epigenetic inactivation of SFRP genes allows constitutive WNT signaling in colorectal cancer. *Nat. Genet.* 2004; 36: 417-422.

[64] Dammann, R., Li, C., Yoon, J. H., Chin, P. L., Bates, S., Pfeifer, G. P. Epigenetic inactivation of a RAS association domain family protein from the lung tumour suppressor locus 3p21.3. *Nat. Genet.* 2000; 25: 315-319.

[65] Bird, A. DNA methylation patterns and epigenetic memory. *Genes Dev.* 2002; 16:6-21.

[66] Wade, P. A. Methyl CpG-binding proteins and transcriptional repression. *Bioessays.* 2001; 23:1131-1137.

[67] Ballestar, E., Wolffe, A. P. Methyl-CpG-binding proteins. Targeting specific gene repression. *Eur. J. Biochem.* 2001; 268:1-6.

[68] Yu, F., Thiesen, J., Stratling, W. H. Histone deacetylase-independent transcriptional repression by methyl-CpG-binding protein 2. *Nucleic Acids Res.* 2000;28:2201-2206.

[69] Kouzarides, T. Histone methylation in transcriptional control. *Curr. Opin. Genet. Dev.* 2002; 12:198-209.

[70] Ropero, S., Fraga, M. F., Ballestar, E., Hamelin, R., Yamamoto, H., Boix-Chornet, M., Caballero, R., Alaminos, M., Setien, F., Paz, M. F., Herranz, M., Palacios, J., Arango, D., Orntoft, T. F., Aaltonen, L. A., Schwartz, S. Jr, Esteller, M. A truncating mutation of HDAC2 in human cancers confers resistance to histone deacetylase inhibition. *Nat. Genet.* 2006; 38:566–569.

[71] Zhu, P., Martin, E., Mengwasser, J., Schlag, P., Janssen, K. P., Göttlicher, M. Induction of HDAC2 expression upon loss of APC in colorectal tumorigenesis. *Cancer Cell.* 2004; 5:455–463.

[72] Lucio-Eterovic, A. K., Cortez, M. A., Valera, E. T., Motta, F. J., Queiroz, R. G., Machado, H. R., Carlotti, C. G. Jr, Neder, L., Scrideli, C. A., Tone, L. G. Differential expression of 12 histone deacetylase (HDAC) genes in astrocytomas and normal brain tissue: class II and IV are hypoexpressed in glioblastomas. *BMC Cancer.* 2008; 8:243.

[73] Isharwal, S., Miller, M. C., Marlow, C., Makarov, D. V., Partin, A. W., Veltri, R. W. p300 (histone acetyltransferase) biomarker predicts prostate cancer biochemical recurrence and correlates with changes in epithelia nuclear size and shape. *Prostate.* 2008; 68:1097–1104.

[74] Roberts, C. W., Orkin, S. H. The SWI/SNF complex-chromatin and cancer. *Nat. Rev. Cancer.* 2004; 4:133-142.

[75] Reisman, D., Glaros, S., Thompson, E. A. The SWI/SNF complex and cancer. *Oncogene.* 2009; 28:1653-1668.

[76] Jones, S., Wang, T. L., Shih IeM, Mao, T. L., Nakayama, K., Roden, R., Glas, R., Slamon, D., Diaz, L. A. Jr, Vogelstein, B., Kinzler, K. W., Velculescu, V. E., Papadopoulos, N. Frequent mutations of chromatin remodeling gene ARID1A in ovarian clear cell carcinoma. *Science.* 2010; 330(6001):228-231.

[77] Lopez, J., Percharde, M., Coley, H. M., Webb, A., Crook, T. The context and potential of epigenetics in oncology. *Br. J. Cancer.* 2009; 100:571–577.

[78] Schickel, R., Boyerinas, B., Park, S. M., Peter, M. E. MicroRNAs: key players in the immune system, differentiation, tumorigenesis and cell death. *Oncogene.* 2008; 27: 5959–5974.

[79] Iorio, M. V., Visone, R., Di Leva, G., Donati, V., Petrocca, F., Casalini, P., Taccioli, C., Volinia, S., Liu, C. G., Alder, H., Calin, G. A., Me´nard, S., Croce, C. M. MicroRNA signatures in human ovarian cancer. *Cancer Res.* 2007; 67:8699–8707.

[80] Schaefer, A., Jung, M., Kristiansen, G., Lein, M., Schrader, M., Miller, K. and Stephan, C., Jung, K. MicroRNAs and cancer: current state and future perspectives in urologic oncology. *Urol. Oncol.* 2010; 28(1):4–13.

[81] Sun, R. P., Fu, X. P., Li, Y., Xie, Y., Mao, Y. M. Global gene expression analysis reveals reduced abundance of putative microRNA targets in human prostate tumors. *BMC Genomics*. 2009; 10:93.

[82] Santarpia, L., Nicoloso, M., Calin, G. A., MicroRNAs: a complex regulatory network drives the acquisition of malignant cell phenotype. *Endocr. Relat. Cancer*. 2009; 17(1): F51–75.

[83] Rigoutsos, I. New tricks for animal microRNAS: targeting of amino acid coding regions at conserved and nonconserved sites. *Cancer Res*. 2009; 69:3245–3248.

[84] Hayashita, Y., Osada, H., Tatematsu, Y., Yamada, H., Yanagisawa, K., Tomida, S., Yatabe, Y., Kawahara, K., Sekido, Y., Takahashi, T. A polycistronic microRNA cluster, miR-17-92, is overexpressed in human lung cancers and enhances cell proliferation. *Cancer Res*. 2005; 65: 9628–9632.

[85] Liang, R. Q., Bates, D. J., Wang, E. Epigenetic control of microRNA expression and aging. *Curr. Genomics*. 2009; 10:184–193.

[86] Visone, R., Russo, L., Pallante, P., De Martino, I., Ferraro, A., Leone, V., Borbone, E., Petrocca, F., Alder, H., Croce, C. M., Fusco, A. MicroRNAs (miR)-221 and miR-222, both overexpressed in human thyroid papillary carcinomas, regulate p27Kip1 protein levels and cell cycle. *Endocr. Relat. Cancer*. 2007; 14:791–798.

[87] Le Sage, C., Nagel, R., Egan, D. A., Schrier, M., Mesman, E., Mangiola, A., Anile, C., Maira, G., Mercatelli, N., Ciafrè, S. A., Farace, M. G., Agami, R. Regulation of the p27(Kip1) tumor suppressor by miR-221 and miR-222 promotes cancer cell proliferation. *EMBO J*. 2007; 26:3699–3708.

[88] Pillai, R. S., Bhattacharyya, S. N., Artus, C. G., Zoller, T., Cougot, N., Basyuk, E., Bertrand, E., Filipowicz, W. Inhibition of translational initiation by Let-7 MicroRNA in human cells. *Science*. 2005; 309:1573–1576.

[89] Chang, S. S., Jiang, W. W., Smith, I., Poeta, L. M., Begum, S., Glazer, C., Shan, S., Westra, W., Sidransky, D., Califano, J. A. MicroRNA alterations in head and neck squamous cell carcinoma. *Int. J. Cancer*. 2008; 123:2791-2797.

[90] Boyerinas, B., Park, S. M., Hau, A., Murmann, A. E., Peter, M. E. The role of let-7 in cell differentiation and cancer. *Endocr. Relat. Cancer*. 2010; 17:F19-F36.

[91] Brueckner, B., Stresemann, C., Kuner, R., Mund, C., Musch, T., Meister, M., Sültmann, H., Lyko, F. The human let-7a-3 locus contains an epigenetically regulated microRNA gene with oncogenic function. *Cancer Res*. 2007; 67:1419-1423.

[92] Krichevsky, A. M., Gabriely, G. miR-21: a small multi-faceted RNA. *J. Cell Mol. Med*. 2009; 13:39-53.

[93] Cimmino, A., Calin, G. A., Fabbri, M., Iorio, M. V., Ferracin, M., Shimizu, M., Wojcik, S. E., Aqeilan, R. I., Zupo, S., Dono, M., Rassenti, L., Alder, H., Volinia, S., Liu, C. G., Kipps, T. J., Negrini, M., Croce, C. M. miR-15 and miR-16 induce apoptosis by targeting BCL2. *Proc. Natl. Acad. Sci. US* 2005; 102:13944-13949.

[94] Tsai, W. C., Hsu, P. W., Lai, T. C., Chau, G. Y., Lin, C. W., Chen, C. M., Lin, C. D., Liao, Y. L., Wang, J. L., Chau, Y. P., Hsu, M. T., Hsiao, M., Huang, H. D., Tsou, A. P. MicroRNA-122, a tumor suppressor microRNA that regulates intrahepatic metastasis of hepatocellular carcinoma. *Hepatology*. 2009; 49:1571-1582.

[95] Le, X. F., Merchant, O., Bast, R. C., Calin, G. A. The roles of microRNAs in the cancer invasion-metastasis cascade. *Cancer Microenviron*. 2010; 3:137-147.

[96] Zhang, B., Pan, X., Cobb, G. P., Anderson, T. A. microRNAs as oncogenes and tumor suppressors. *Dev. Biol.* 2007; 302:1-12.

[97] Ma, L., Weinberg, R. A. Micromanagers of malignancy: role of microRNAs in regulating metastasis. *Trends Genet.* 2008; 24:448-456.

[98] O'Day, E., Lal, A. MicroRNAs and their target gene networks in breast cancer. *Breast Cancer Res.* 2010; 12:201.

[99] Passetti, F., Ferreira, C. G., Costa, F. F. The impact of microRNAs and alternative splicing in pharmacogenomics. *Pharmacogenomics J.* 2009; 9:1–13.

[100] Iorio, M. V., Croce, C. M. MicroRNAs in cancer: small molecules with a huge impact. *J. Clin. Oncol.* 2009; 27:5848–5856.

[101] Jemal, A., Siegel, R., Ward, E., Hao, Y. P., Xu, J. Q., Thun, M. J. Cancer statistics, 2009. *CA Cancer J. Clin.* 2009; 59:225–249.

[102] Chen, Z., Wang, L., Wang, Q., Li, W. Histone modifications and chromatin organization in prostate cancer. *Epigenomics.* 2010; 2(4):551-560.

[103] Kang, Z., Janne, O. A., Palvimo, J. J. Coregulator recruitment and histone modifications in transcriptional regulation by the androgen receptor. *Mol. Endocrinol.* 2004; 18(11):2633–2648.

[104] Yu, J., Cao, Q., Mehra, R., Laxman, B., Yu, J., Tomlins, S. A., Creighton, C. J., Dhanasekaran, S. M., Shen, R., Chen, G., Morris, D. S., Marquez, V. E., Shah, R. B., Ghosh, D., Varambally, S., Chinniyan, A. M. Integrative genomics analysis reveals silencing of β-adrenergic signaling by polycomb in prostate cancer. *Cancer Cell.* 2007; 12(5): 419–431.

[105] Cao, R., Zhang, Y. The functions of E(Z)/EZH2-mediated methylation of lysine 27 in histone H3. *Curr. Opin. Genet. Dev.* 2004; 14(2):155–164.

[106] Varambally, S., Dhanasekaran, S. M., Zhou, M., Baretta, T. R., Kumar-Sinha, C., Sanda, M. G., Ghosh, D., Pienta, K. J., Sewalt, R. G., Otte, A. P., Rubin, M. A., Chinnaiyan, A. M. The polycomb group protein EZH2 is involved in progression of prostate cancer. *Nature.* 2002; 419 (6907): 624–629.

[107] Kondo, Y., Shen, L., Chenq, A. S., Ahmed, S., Boumber, Y., Charo, C., Yamochi, T., Urano, T., Furukawa, K., Kwabi-Addo, B., Gold, D. L., Sekido, Y., Huanq, T. H., Issa, J. P. Gene silencing in cancer by histone H3 lysine 27 trimethylation independent of promoter DNA methylation. *Nat. Genet.* 2008; 40(6):741–750.

[108] Seligson, D. B., Horvath, S., Shi, T., Yu, H., Tze, S., Grunstein, M., Kurdistani, S. K. Global histone modification patterns predict risk of prostate cancer recurrence. *Nature.* 2005; 435(7046):1262–1266.

[109] Fullwood, M. J., Liu, M. H., Pan, Y. F., Liu, J., Xu, H., Mohamed, Y. B., Orlov, Y. L., Velkov, S., Ho, A., Mei, P. H., Chew, E. G., Huang, P. Y., Welboren, W. J., Han, Y., Ooi, H. S, Ariyaratne, P. N., Vega, V. B., Luo, Y., Tan, P. Y., Choy, P. Y., Wansa, K. D., Zhao, B., Lim, K. S., Leow, S. C., Yow, J. S., Joseph, R., Li, H., Desai, K. V., Thomsen, J. S., Lee, Y. K., Karutiri, R. K., Herve, T., Bourque, G., Stunnenberg, H. G., Ruan, X., Cacheux-Rataboul, V., Sung, W. K., Liu, E. T., Wei, C. L., Cheung, E., Ruan, Y. An oestrogen-receptor-α-bound human chromatin interactome. *Nature.* 2009; 462(7269):58–64.

[110] Kouzarides, T. Chromatin modifications and their function. *Cell.* 2007; 128(4):693–705.

[111] Martin, C., Zhang, Y. The diverse functions of histone lysine methylation. *Nat. Rev. Mol. Cell Biol.* 2005; 6(11):838–849.

[112] Vrba, L., Jensen, T. J., Garbe, J. C., Heimark, R. L., Cress, A. E., Dickinson, S., Stampfer, M. R., Futscher, B. W. Role for DNA methylation in the regulation of miR-200c and miR-141 expression in normal and cancer cells. *PLoS One.* 2010; 5(1):e8697.

[113] Mattie, M. D., Benz, C. C., Bowers, J., Sensinger, K., Wong, L., Scott, G. K., and Fedele, V., Ginzinger, D., Getts, R., Haqq, C. Optimized high-throughput microRNA expression profiling provides novel biomarker assessment of clinical prostate and breast cancer biopsies. *Mol. Cancer.* 2006; 5:24.

[114] Porkka, K. P., Pfeiffer, M. J., Waltering, K. K., Vessella, R. L., Tammela, T. L., and Visakorpi, T. MicroRNA expression profiling in prostate cancer. *Cancer Res.* 2007; 67: 6130–6135.

[115] Ribas, J., Ni, X. H., Haffner, M., Wentzel, E. A., Salmasi, A. H., Chowdhury, W. H., Kudrolli, T. A., Yeqnasubramanian, S., Luo, J., Rodriquez, R., Mendell, J. T., Lupold, S. E. miR-21: an androgen receptor-regulated microRNA that promotes hormone-dependent and hormone-independent prostate cancer growth. *Cancer Res.* 2009; 69: 7165–7169.

[116] Mercatelli, N., Coppola, V., Bonci, D., Miele, F., Costantini, A., Guadagnoli, M., and Bonanno, E., Muto, G., Frajese, G. V., De Maria, R., Spagnoli, L. G., Farace, M. G., Ciafre, S. A. The inhibition of the highly expressed miR-221 and miR-222 impairs the growth of prostate carcinoma xenografts in mice. *PLoS One.* 2008; 3(12):e4029.

[117] Li, T., Li, D., Sha, J. J., Sun, P., Huang, Y. R. MicroRNA-21 directly targets MARCKS and promotes apoptosis resistance and invasion in prostate cancer cells. *Biochem. Biophys. Res. Commun.* 2009; 383:280–285.

[118] Lee, Y. S., Kim, H. K., Chung, S., Kim, K. S., and Dutta, A. Depletion of human micro-RNA miR-125b reveals that it is critical for the proliferation of differentiated cells but not for the down-regulation of putative targets during differentiation. *J. Biol. Chem.* 2005; 280:16635-16641.

[119] Musiyenko, A., Bitko, V., Barik, S. Ectopic expression of miR-126*, an intronic product of the vascular endothelial EGF-like 7 gene, regulates prostein translation and invasiveness of prostate cancer LNCaP cells. *J. Mol. Med.* 2008; 86:313-322.

[120] Lin, S. L., Chiang, A., Chang, D., Ying, S. Y. Loss of mir-146a function in hormone-refractory prostate cancer. *RNA.* 2008; 14:417-424.

[121] Lee, K. H., Chen, Y. L., Yeh, S. D., Hsiao, M., Lin, J. T., Goan, Y. G., Lu, P. J. MicroRNA-330 acts as tumor suppressor and induces apoptosis of prostate cancer cells through E2F1-mediated suppression of Akt phosphorylation. *Oncogene.* 2009; 28:3360-3370.

[122] Rokhlin, O. W., Scheinker, V. S., Taghiyev, A. F., Bumcrot, D., Glover, R. A., Cohen, M. B. MicroRNA-34 mediates AR-dependent p53-induced apoptosis in prostate cancer. *Cancer Biol. Ther.* 2008; 7:1288-1296.

[123] Arai, E., Kanai, Y. Genetic and epigenetic alterations during renal carcinogenesis. *Int. J. Clin. Exp. Pathol.* 2011; 4(1):58-73.

[124] Liang, S., Xu, Y., Shen, G., Zhao, X., Zhou, J., Li, X., Gong, F., Ling, B., Fang, L., Huang, C., Wei, Y. Gene expression and methylation status of 14-3-3sigma in human renal carcinoma tissues. *IUBMB Life.* 2008; 60:534-540.

[125] To, K. K., Zhan, Z., Bates, S. E. Aberrant promoter methylation of the ABCG2 gene in renal carcinoma. *Mol. Cell Biol.* 2006; 26:8572-8585.

[126] Yano, T., Ito, F., Kobayashi, K., Yonezawa, Y., Suzuki, K., Asano, R., Hagiwara, K., Nakazawa, H., Toma, H., Yamasaki, H. Hypermethylation of the CpG island of connexin 32, a candiate tumor suppressor gene in renal cell carcinomas from hemodialysis patients. *Cancer Lett.* 2004; 208:137-142.

[127] Yamada, D., Kikuchi, S., Williams, Y. N., Sakurai-Yageta, M., Masuda, M., Maruyama, T., Tomita, K., Gutmann, D. H., Kakizoe, T., Kitamura, T., Kanai, Y., Murakami, Y. Promoter hypermethylation of the potential tumor suppressor DAL-1/4.1B gene in renal clear cell carcinoma. *Int. J. Cancer.* 2006; 118:916-923.

[128] Onay, H., Pehlivan, S., Koyuncuoglu, M., Kirkali, Z., and Ozkinay, F. Multigene methylation analysis of conventional renal cell carcinoma. *Urol. Int.* 2009; 83:107-112.

[129] Kvasha, S., Gordiyuk, V., Kondratov, A., Ugryn, D., Zgonnyk, Y. M., Rynditch, A. V., and Vozianov, A. F. Hypermethylation of the 5'CpG island of the FHIT gene in clear cell renal carcinomas. *Cancer Lett.* 2008; 265:250-257.

[130] Breault, J. E., Shiina, H., Igawa, M., Ribeiro-Filho, L. A., Deguchi, M., Enokida, H., Urakami, S., Terashima, M., Nakagawa, M., Kane, C. J., Carroll, P. R., Dahiya, R. Methylation of the gamma-catenin gene is associated with poor prognosis of renal cell carcinoma. *Clin. Cancer Res.* 2005; 11:557-564.

[131] Morris, M. R., Gentle, D., Abdulrahman, M., Maina, E. N., Gupta, K., Banks, R. E., Wiesener, M. S., Kishida, T., Yao, M., The, B., Latif, F., Maher, E. R. Tumor suppressor activity and epigenetic inactivation of hepatocyte growth factor activator inhibitor type 2/SPINT2 in papillary and clear renal cell carcinoma. *Cancer Res.* 2055; 65(11):4598-606.

[132] Okuda, H., Toyota, M., Ishida, W., Furihata, M., Tsuchiya, M., Kamada, M., Tokino, T., Shuin, T. Epigenetic inactivation of the candidate tumor suppressor gene HOXB13 in human renal cell carcinoma. *Oncogene.* 2006; 25:1733-1742.

[133] Sturm, I., Stephan, C., Gillissen, B., Siebert, R., Janz, M., Radetzki, S., Jung, K., Loening, S., Dorken, B., Daniel, P. T. Loss of the tissue-specific proapoptotic BH3-only protein Nbk/Bik is a unifying feature of renal cell carcinoma. *Cell Death Differ.* 2006; 13:619-627.

[134] Awakura, Y., Nakamura, E., Ito, N., Kamoto, T., Ogawa, O. Methylation-associated silencing of TU3A in human cancers. *Int. J. Oncol.* 2008; 33:893-899.

[135] Kempkensteffen, C., Hinz, S., Schrader, M., Christoph, F., Magheli, A., Krause, H., Schostak, M., Miller, K., Weikert, S. Gene expression and promoter methylation of the XIAP-associated Factor 1 in renal cell carcinomas: correlations with pathology and outcome. *Cancer Lett.* 2007; 254:227-235.

[136] McRonald, F. E., Morris, M. R., Gentle, D., Winchester, L., Baban, D., Ragoussis, J., Clarke, N. W., Brown, M. D., Kishida, T., Yao, M., Latif, F., Maher, E. R. CpG methylation profiling in VHL related and VHL unrelated renal cell carcinoma. *Mol. Cancer.* 2009; 8:31.

[137] Urakami, S., Shiina, H., Enokida, H., Hirata, H., Kawamoto, K., Kawakami, T., Kikuno, N., Tanaka, Y., Majid, S., Nakagawa, M., Igawa, M., Dahiya, R. Wnt antagonist family genes as biomarkers for diagnosis, staging, and prognosis of renal cell carcinoma using tumor and serum DNA. *Clin. Cancer Res.* 2006; 12:6989-6997.

[138] Kagara, I., Enokida, H., Kawakami, K., Matsuda, R., Toki, K., Nishimura, H., Chiyomaru, T., Tatarano, S., Itesako, T., Kawamoto, K., Nishiyama, K., Seki, N., Nakagawa, M. CpG hypermethylation of the UCHL1 gene promoter is associated with pathogenesis and poor prognosis in renal cell carcinoma. *J. Urol.* 2008; 180:343-351.

[139] Cho, M., Uemura, H., Kim, S. C., Kawada, Y., Yoshida, K., Hirao, Y., Konishi, N., Saga, S., Yoshikawa, K. Hypomethylation of the MN/CA9 promoter and upregulated MN/CA9 expression in human renal cell carcinoma. *Br. J. Cancer.* 2001; 85:563-567.

[140] Jung, M., Mollenkopf, H. J., Grimm, C., Wagner, I., Albrecht, M., Waller, T., Pilarsky, C., Johannsen, M., Stephan, C., Lehrach, H., Nietfeld, W., Rudel, T., Jung, K., Kristiansen, G. MicroRNA profiling of clear cell renal cell cancer identifies a robust signature to define renal malignancy. *J. Cell Mol. Med.* 2009; 13:3918–3928.

[141] Nakada, C., Matsuura, K., Tsukamoto, Y., Tanigawa, M., Yoshimoto, T., Narimatsu, T., Nguyen, L. T., Hijiya, N., Uchida, T., Sato, F., Mimata, H., Seto, M., Moriyama, M. Genome-wide microRNA expression profiling in renal cell carcinoma: significant down-regulation of miR-141 and miR-200c. *J. Pathol.* 2008; 216:418-427.

[142] Dulaimi, E., Uzzo, R. G., Greenberg, R. E., Al-Saleem, T., Cairns, P. Detection of bladder cancer in urine by a tumor suppressor gene hypermethylation panel. *Clin. Cancer Res.* 2004; 10:1887-1893.

[143] Esteller, M., Hamilton, S. R., Burger, P. C., Baylin, S. B., Herman, J. G. Inactivation of the DNA repair gene O6-methylguanine-DNA methyltransferase by promoter hypermethylation is a common event in primary human neoplasia. *Cancer Res.* 1999; 59:793–797.

[144] Mori, K., Enokida, H., Kagara, I., Kawakami, K., Chiyomaru, T., Tatarano, S., Kawahara, K., Nishiyama, K., Seki, N., Nakaqawa, M. CpG hypermethylation of collagen type I alpha 2 contributes to proliferation and migration activity of human bladder cancer. *Int. J. Oncol.* 2009; 34:1593-1602.

[145] Liang, G., Gonzales, F. A., Jones, P. A., Orntoft, T. F., Thykjaer, T. Analysis of gene induction in human fibroblasts and bladder cancer cells exposed to the methylation inhibitor 5-aza-2'-deoxycytidine. *Cancer Res.* 2002; 62:961-966.

[146] Wu, G., Guo, Z., Chang, X., Kim, M. S., Nagpal, J. K., Liu, J., Maki, J. M., Kivirikko, K. I., Ethier, S. P., Trink, B., Sidransky, D. LOXL1 and LOXL4 are epigenetically silenced and can inhibit ras/ extracellular signal-regulated kinase signaling pathway in human bladder cancer. *Cancer Res.* 2007; 67:4123-4129.

[147] Veerla, S., Panagopoulos, I., Jin, Y., Lindgren, D., Hoglund, M. Promoter analysis of epigenetically controlled genes in bladder cancer. *Genes Chromosomes Cancer.* 2008; 47:368-378.

[148] Nguyen, C. T., Weisenberger, D. J., Velicescu, M., Gonzales, F. A., Lin, J. C., Liang, G., Jones, P. A. Histone H3-lysine 9 methylation is associated with aberrant gene silencing in cancer cells and is rapidly reversed by 5-aza-2'-deoxycytidine. *Cancer Res.* 2002; 62:6456-6461.

[149] Campan, M., Weisenberger, D. J., Laird, P. W. DNA methylation profiles of female steroid hormone-driven human malignancies. *Curr. Top Microbiol. Immunol.* 2006; 310:141-178.

[150] Yanokura, M., Banno, K., Susumu, N., Kawaguchi, M., Kuwabara, Y., Tsukazaki, K., Aoki, D. Hypermethylation in the p16 promoter region in the carcinogenesis of endometrial cancer in Japanese patients. *Anticancer Res.* 2006; 26(2A):851-856.

[151] Whitcomb, B. P., Mutch, D. G., Herzog, T. J., Rader, J. S., Gibb, R. K., Goodfellow, P. J. Frequent HOXA11 and THBS2 promoter methylation and a methylator phenotype in endometrial adenocarcinoma. *Clin. Cancer Res.* 2003; 9(6):2277-2287.

[152] Yeh, K. T., Yang, M. Y., Liu, T. C., Chen, J. C., Chan, W. L., Lin, S. F., Chang, J. G. Abnormal expression of period 1 (PER1) in endometrial carcinoma. *J. Pathol.* 2005; 206(1):111-120.

[153] Gurin, C. C., Federici, M. G., Kang, L., Boyd, J. Causes and consequences of microsatellite instability in endometrial carcinoma. *Cancer Res.* 1999; 59(2):462-466.

[154] Jacinto, F. V., Esteller, M. Mutator pathways unleashed by epigenetic silencing in human cancer. *Mutagenesis.* 2007; 22(4):247-253.

[155] Balch, C., Matei, D., Huang, T., Nephew, K. P. Role of epigenomics in ovarian and endometrial cancers. *Epigenomics.* 2010; 2(3):419-447.

[156] Izutsu, N., Maesawa, C., Shibazaki, M., Oikawa, H., Shoji, T., Suqiyama, T., Masuda, T. Epigenetic modification is involved in aberrant expression of class III b-tubulin, TUBB3, in ovarian cancer cells. *Int. J. Oncol.* 2008; 32(6);1227-1235.

[157] Press, J. Z., De Luca, A., Boyd, N., Young, S., Troussard, A., Ridge, Y., Kaurah, P., Kalloger, S. E., Blood, K. A., Smith, M., Spellman, P. T., Wang, Y., Miller, D. M., Horsman, D., Faham, M., Gilks, C. B., Gray, J., Huntsman, D. G. Ovarian carcinomas with genetic and epigenetic BRCA1 loss have distinct molecular abnormalities. *BMC Cancer.* 2008; 8:17.

[158] Milde-Langosch, K., Ocon, E., Becker, G., Löning, T. p16/MTS1 inactivation in ovarian carcinomas: high frequency of reduced protein expression associated with hyper-methylation or mutation in endometrioid and mucinous tumors. *Int. J. Cancer.* 1998; 79:61-65.

[159] Ibanezde Caceres, I., Battagli, C., Esteller, M., Herman, J. G., Dulaimi, E., Edelson, M. I., Bergman, C., Ehya, H., Eisenberg, B. L., Cairns, P. Tumor cell-specific BRCA1 and RASSF1A hypermethylation in serum, plasma, and peritoneal fluid from ovarian cancer patients. *Cancer Res.* 2004; 64:6476-6481.

[160] Cvetkovic, D., Pisarcik, D., Lee, C., Hamilton, T. C., Abdollahi, A. Altered expression and loss of heterozygosity of the LOT1 gene in ovarian cancer. *Gynecol. Oncol.* 2004; 95:449-455.

[161] Terasawa, K., Sagae, S., Toyota, M., Tsukada, K., Ogi, K., Satoh, A., Mita, H., Imai, K., Tokino, T., Kudo, R. Epigenetic inactivation of TMS1/ASC in ovarian cancer. *Clin. Cancer Res.* 2004; 10:2000-2006.

[162] Yuecheng, Y., Hongmei, L., Xiaoyan, X. Clinical evaluation of E-cadherin expression and its regulation mechanism in epithelial ovarian cancer. *Clin. Exp. Metastasis.* 2006; 23:65-74.

[163] Backen, A. C., Cole, C. L., Lau, S. C., Clamp, A. R., McVey, R., Gallagher, J. T., Jayson, G. C. Heparan sulphate synthetic and editing enzymes in ovarian cancer. *Br. J. Cancer.* 2007; 96:1544-1548Dd.

[164] Staub, J., Chien, J., Pan, Y., Qian, X., Narita, K., Aletti, G., Scheerer, M., Roberts, L. R., Molina, J., Shridhar, V. Epigenetic silencing of HSulf-1 in ovarian cancer: implications in chemoresistance. *Oncogene.* 2007; 26:4969-4978.

[165] Potapova, A., Hoffman, A. M., Godwin, A. K., Al-Saleem, T., Cairns, P. Promoter hypermethylation of the PALB2 susceptibility gene in inherited and sporadic breast and ovarian cancer. *Cancer Res.* 2008; 68:998-1002.

[166] Murphy, S. K., Huang, Z., Wen, Y., Spillman, M. A., Whitaker, R. S., Simel, L. R., Nichols, T. D., Marks, J. R., Berchuck, A. Frequent IGF2/H19 domain epigenetic alterations and elevated IGF2 expression in epithelial ovarian cancer. *Mol. Cancer Res.* 2006; 4(4):283–292.

[167] Litkouhi, B., Kwong, J., Lo, C. M., Smedley, 3rd J. G., McClane, B. A., Aponte, M., Gao, Z., Sarno, J. L., Hinners, J., Welch, W. R., Berkowitz, R. S., Mok, S. C., Garner, E. I. Claudin-4 overexpression in epithelial ovarian cancer is associated with hypomethylation and is a potential target for modulation of tight junction barrier function using a C-terminal fragment of Clostridium perfringens enterotoxin. *Neoplasia.* 2007; 9(4):304-314.

[168] Pattamadilok, J., Huapai, N., Rattanatanyong, P., Vasurattana, A., Triratanachat, S., Tresukosal, D., Mutirangura, A. LINE-1 hypomethylation level as a potential prognostic factor for epithelial ovarian cancer. *Int. J. Gynecol Cancer.* 2008; 18(4):711-717.

[169] Bram, E. E., Stark, M., Raz, S., Assaraf, Y. G. Chemotherapeutic drug-induced ABCG2 promoter demethylation as a novel mechanism of acquired multidrug resistance. *Neoplasia.* 2009; 11(12):1359-1370.

[170] Honda, H., Pazin, M. J., D'Souza, T., Ji, H., Morin, P. J. Regulation of the CLDN3 gene in ovarian cancer cells. *Cancer Biol. Ther.* 2007; 6(11); 1733-1742.

[171] Strathdee, G., Vass, J. K., Oien, K. A., Siddiqui, N., Curto-Garcia, J., Brown, R. Demethylation of the MCJ gene in stage III/IV epithelial ovarian cancer and response to chemotherapy. *Gynecol. Oncol.* 2005; 97: 898-903.

[172] LaVoie, H. A. Epigenetic control of ovarian function: the emerging role of histone modifications. *Mol. Cell Endocrinol.* 2005; 243:12-18.

[173] Chan, M. W., Huang, Y. W., Hartman-Frey, C., Kuo, C. T., Deatherage, D., Qin, H., Cheng, A. S., Yan, P. S., Davuluri, R. V., Huang, T. H., Nephew, K. P., Lin, H. J. Aberrant transforming growth factor-1 signaling and SMAD4 nuclear translocation confer epigenetic repression of ADAM19 in ovarian cancer. *Neoplasia.* 2008; 10:908-919.

[174] Wei, Y., Xia, W., Zhang, Z., Liu, J., Wang, H., Adsay, N. V., Albarracin, C., Yu, D., Abbruzzese, J. L., Mills, G. B., Bast, Jr R. C., Hortobagyi GN, Hung MC. Loss of trimethylation at lysine 27 of histone H3 is a predictor of poor outcome in breast, ovarian, and pancreatic cancers. *Mol. Carcinog.* 2008; 47:701-706.

[175] Weichert, W., Denkert, C., Noske, A., Darb-Esfahani, S., Dietel, M., Kalloger, S. E., Huntsman, D. G., Köbel, M. Expression of class I histone deacetylases indicates poor prognosis in endometrioid subtypes of ovarian and endometrial carcinomas. *Neoplasia.* 2008; 10(9):1021-1027.

[176] Parekh, D. J., Ankerst, D. P., Troyer, D., Srivastava, S., Thompson, I. M. Biomarkers for prostate cancer detection. *J. Urol.* 2007; 178:2252-2259.

[177] Zhang, L., Volinia, S., Bonome, T., Calin, G. A., Greshock, J., Yang, N., Liu, C. G., Giannakakis, A., Alexiou, P., Hasegawa, K., Johnstone, C. N., Megraw, M. S., Adams, S., Lassus, H., Huang, J., Kaur, S., Liang, S., Sethupathy, P., Leminen, A., Simossis, V. A., Sandaltzopoulos, R., Naomoto, Y., Katsaros, D., Gimotty, P. A., DeMichele, A., Huang, Q., Bützow, R., Rustgi, A. K., Weber, B. L., Birrer, M. J., Hatzigeorgiou, A. G., Croce, C. M., Coukos G. Genomic and epigenetic alterations deregulate microRNA

expression in human epithelial ovarian cancer. *Proc. Natl. Acad. Sci. US* 2008; 105(19): 7004-7009.

[178] Shankar, S., Srivastava, R. K. Histone Deacetylase Inhibitors: Mechanisms and clinical significance in cancer. Khrosravi-Far R, White E. *Programmed Cell Death in Cancer Progression and Therapy.* Springer. 2008; 261-298.

Index

E

N